Keto Diet Cookbook for Beginners

2000 Days of Quick and Easy Low-Carb Recipes with a 30-Day Meal Plan for Busy People Who Want to Lose Weight and Stay Healthy"

Adopt a Healthier Lifestyle Without Giving Up Great Taste

Isabella Carr

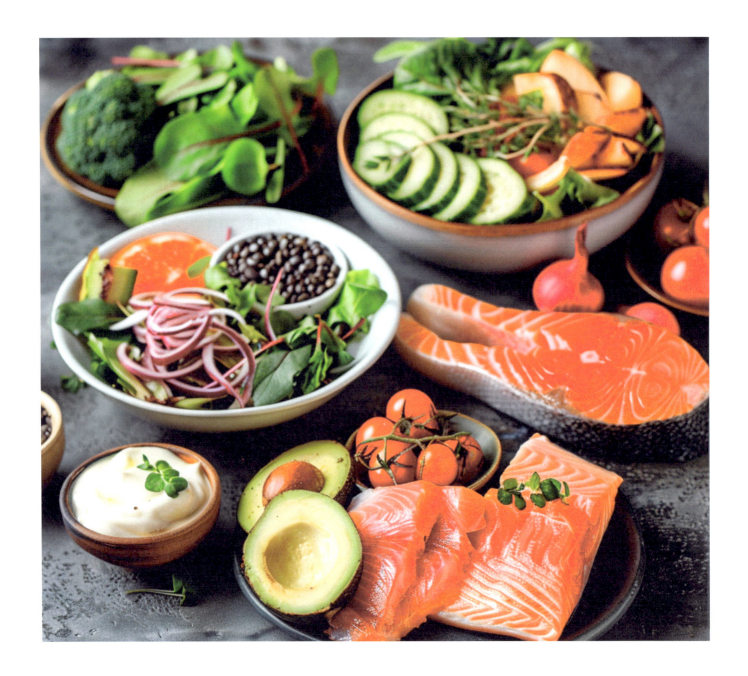

TABLE OF CONTENTS

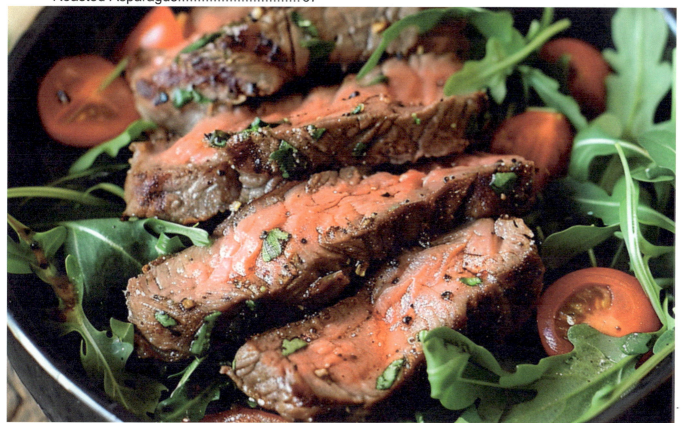

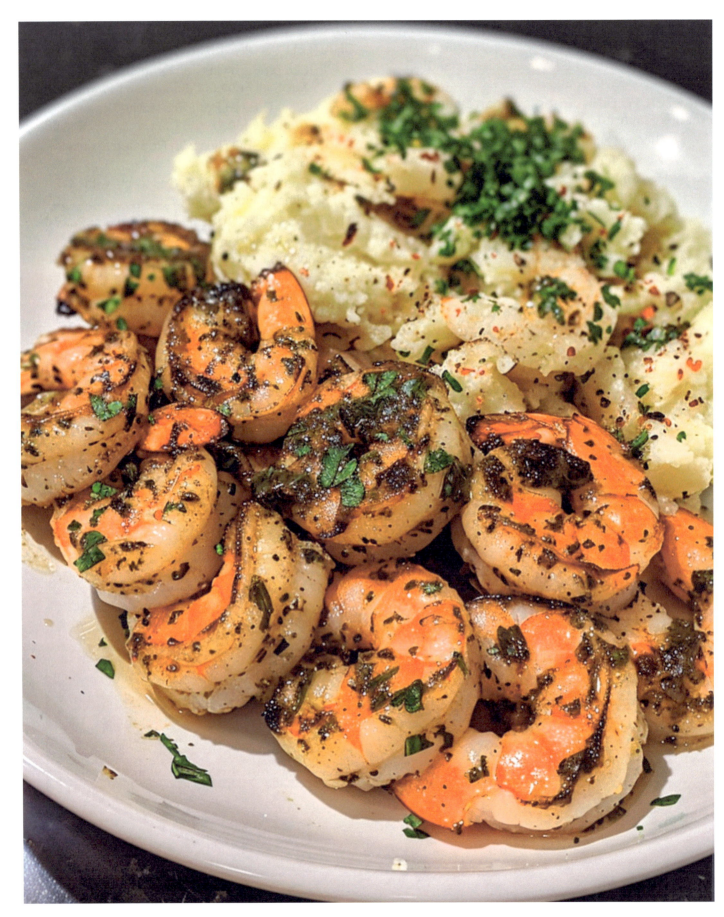

INTRODUCTION

Dear readers,

Isabella Carr, a renowned chef specializing in keto cuisine, introduces her book, ***"Keto Diet Cookbook for Beginners."*** Drawing from her extensive culinary background, **Isabella** has mastered the creation of meals that are both delicious and perfectly suited to the ketogenic lifestyle.

In this cookbook, **Isabella** combines her professional expertise with a passion for health-focused cooking. Each recipe is crafted to be easy to prepare, nutrient-dense, and optimized to support weight management and sustained energy. Understanding the challenges of starting keto, **Isabella** provides practical guidance and accessible solutions to make the journey effortless.

The book features a 30-day meal plan designed to help beginners embrace the keto diet with ease. Beyond a collection of recipes, it's a comprehensive guide to creating a sustainable and enjoyable way of eating. Whether you're just starting out or seeking new recipe ideas, **Isabella's** cookbook equips you with everything needed for success.

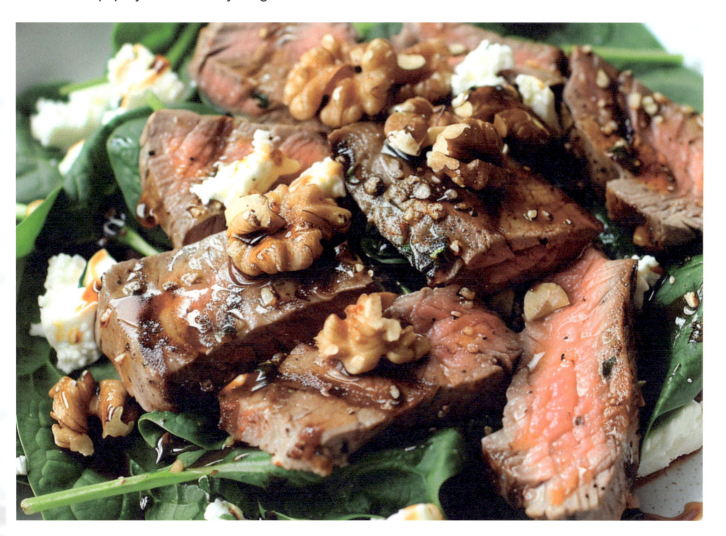

CHAPTER 1: INTRODUCTION TO THE KETO DIET

Welcome to the Keto Journey

The ketogenic lifestyle is far more than a diet—it's a transformative path to enhanced health, sustained energy, and overall vitality. While weight loss often draws the most attention, the true strength of keto lies in its ability to sharpen mental focus, regulate blood sugar, and promote metabolic health—all while indulging in flavorful, satisfying meals.

At its essence, the keto diet emphasizes high-fat, low-carbohydrate eating, guiding your body into a metabolic state called ketosis. In ketosis, fat becomes the primary energy source, replacing glucose. This shift not only speeds up fat burning but also ensures lasting energy, reduces cravings, and optimizes brain function.

Whether you're new to keto or refining your approach, this book serves as your ultimate resource. We'll explain the science behind ketosis, highlight its many advantages, and provide practical steps for adopting and maintaining this lifestyle. From key foods and shopping strategies to expertly crafted recipes, you'll have everything you need to make keto a sustainable and enjoyable part of your life.

As a chef experienced in ketogenic cooking, I've designed this book to help you create meals that are both balanced and bursting with flavor. These recipes and insights will show you that keto isn't about limitation—it's about redefining your relationship with food and transforming your body and health.

Benefits of the Keto Journey

Switching to keto unlocks a host of health benefits that extend far beyond shedding extra pounds. Here's why keto is celebrated worldwide:

1. **Fast Fat Burning**
   By cutting down on carbs, your body enters ketosis, burning fat for fuel. This metabolic shift, paired with reduced insulin levels, promotes rapid and sustainable fat loss.
2. **Clearer Thinking**
   Ketones, the byproducts of fat metabolism, provide clean energy for the brain. Many report sharper focus, better memory, and improved cognitive function, making keto ideal for busy lifestyles.
3. **Steady Energy**
   Unlike carb-heavy diets that cause energy highs and crashes, keto provides a consistent, long-lasting energy supply thanks to fat's efficiency as fuel.
4. **Hunger Control**
   The high-fat, moderate-protein nature of keto meals keeps you satisfied longer, naturally reducing hunger and overeating.
5. **Heart Health**
   Keto can raise HDL (good cholesterol) and lower triglycerides, improving overall cardiovascular health despite its focus on fats.
6. **Balanced Blood Sugar**
   By limiting carbohydrates, keto helps maintain stable blood sugar levels, benefiting those with diabetes or insulin resistance.

7. **Reduced Inflammation**
   Cutting out processed carbs and sugars while increasing healthy fats can lower inflammation, easing joint pain and enhancing overall wellness.
8. **Simplified Lifestyle**
   Keto offers plenty of satisfying options. Meal prep becomes straightforward, and dining out is manageable with minor adjustments.

Understanding Ketosis

What is Ketosis?
Ketosis is a metabolic state where your body relies on fat for energy instead of carbs. This occurs when carb intake is drastically reduced, prompting the liver to produce ketones from fat to fuel the body.

How Ketosis Works:

- **Switching Fuel Sources:** Reducing carbs to 20–50 grams per day depletes glycogen stores, forcing the body to use fat for energy.
- **Ketone Creation:** The liver converts fatty acids into ketones, which fuel the brain, muscles, and other tissues.
- **Fat Burning:** The body efficiently uses dietary and stored fat, leading to weight loss and increased energy.

Signs You're in Ketosis:

- Decreased appetite
- Enhanced focus and clarity
- Steady energy
- Mild acetone-like breath

Maintaining Ketosis:
Consistency is key. Focus on high-fat, moderate-protein, and low-carb meals while avoiding hidden sugars and processed carbs.

Keto-Approved Foods

Healthy Fats:

- Avocados, avocado oil
- Olive oil, coconut oil, MCT oil
- Grass-fed butter, ghee

Proteins:

- Grass-fed beef, pork, and lamb
- Free-range poultry
- Fatty fish such as salmon and sardines
- Eggs

Low-Carb Vegetables:

- Spinach, kale, arugula
- Broccoli, cauliflower, Brussels sprouts
- Zucchini, asparagus, bell peppers

Keto-Friendly Fruits:

- Strawberries, raspberries, blackberries
- Lemons and limes (in moderation)

Dairy Options:

- Full-fat cheeses
- Heavy cream
- Unsweetened almond or coconut milk

Foods to Avoid:

- Sugary snacks and drinks
- Grains like bread, pasta, and rice
- High-carb fruits such as bananas and mangoes
- Starchy vegetables like potatoes
- Legumes including beans and lentils

Managing Keto Flu

The transition to ketosis may cause flu-like symptoms, known as "keto flu." Here's how to ease this process:

1. **Electrolytes:**
   Increase sodium, potassium, and magnesium intake through foods like leafy greens, nuts, and avocados, or consider supplements.
2. **Hydration:**
   Drink plenty of water to prevent dehydration.
3. **Adequate Fats:**
   Consume enough healthy fats to fuel your body during the transition.
4. **Gradual Adjustment:**
   Ease into keto by reducing carbs gradually instead of all at once.
5. **Rest and Recovery:**
   Prioritize sleep and avoid intense exercise during the first week to allow your body to adapt.

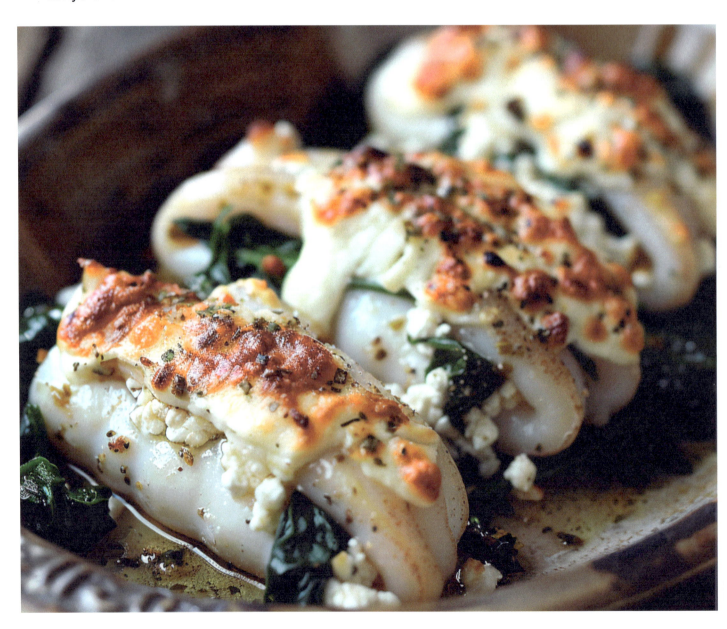

CHAPTER 2: 30-DAY MEAL PLAN

Day	Breakfast	Lunch	Snack	Dinner
Day 1	Smoked Salmon Eggs Benedict with Lemon Hollandaise (p.16)	Creamy Chicken Zucchini Noodle Soup (p.28)	Zucchini Roll-Ups with Herbed Ricotta (p.43)	Garlic Herb Chicken with Roasted Cherry Tomatoes (p.57)
Day 2	Cheddar and Herb Keto Egg Muffins (p.16)	Zucchini Noodle Pad Thai Bowl (p.32)	Lemon Garlic Chicken Skewers (p.42)	Butter-Poached Lobster with Cauliflower Puree (p.66)
Day 3	Ricotta-Stuffed Peppers with Spinach and Basil (p.18)	Keto Thai Coconut Shrimp Soup (p.29)	Baked Jalapeño Poppers with Cheddar Cheese (p.42)	Shrimp Scampi with Lemon Garlic Cauliflower Rice (p.65)
Day 4	Blueberry Antioxidant Shake (p.23)	Creamy Garlic Shirataki Alfredo (p.34)	Coconut Raspberry Chia Pudding (p.47)	Crispy Pork Cutlets with Creamy Dijon Cabbage Slaw (p.58)
Day 5	Family-Style Chorizo Breakfast Bowls (p.25)	Stuffed Bell Peppers with Lamb and Spinach (p.38)	Lemon Dill Yogurt Sauce (p.46)	Grilled Salmon with Lemon Dill Sauce (p.37)
Day 6	Egg Crepe Toast with Bacon and Avocado (p.20)	Pork & Brussels Sprouts Bowl with Garlic Butter (p.32)	Smoked Paprika Mayo with Cheddar Crisps (p.46)	Slow-Cooked Pork Roast with Creamy Cabbage Mash (p.68)
Day 7	Green Detox Spinach Smoothie (p.23)	French Onion Soup with Gruyere Cheese (p.29)	Keto Vanilla Coconut Custard (p.49)	Seared Steak Bites with Garlic Butter Green Beans (p.58)
Day 8	Pesto Mushroom and Bacon Bake (p.15)	Spaghetti Carbonara with Zucchini Noodles (p.34)	Dark Chocolate and Almond Keto Fat Bombs (p.47)	Lemon Chicken with Zucchini Noodles and Capers (p.59)
Day 9	Zucchini and Cheddar Herb Muffins with Thyme (p.22)	Greek Cauliflower Rice Bowl with Chicken and Feta (p.33)	Cinnamon Almond Crumble Bars (p.48)	Mackerel in Lemon Herb Butter with Roasted Asparagus (p.67)
Day 10	Almond Flour Hash Browns with Sour Cream (p.26)	Tomato Basil Keto Soup with Parmesan Chips (p.31)	Crispy Cauliflower Bites with Garlic Aioli (p.43)	Parmesan-Crusted Zucchini Fritters with Lemon Yogurt Sauce (p.56)
Day 11	Avocado and Spinach Power Smoothie (p.24)	Balsamic-Glazed Chicken with Broccoli Mash (p.38)	Strawberry Cream Keto Shortcake (p.52)	Vegan Ratatouille with Olives and Basil (p.64)
Day 12	Greek Egg Bake with Feta, Spinach, and Olives (p.17)	Mushroom and Leek Keto Stew (p.29)	Keto Mocha Layered Bars (p.50)	BBQ Chicken Thighs with Creamy Cabbage Slaw (p.39)
Day 13	Tomato and Egg Cheese Boats (p.20)	Keto Burrito Bowl with Ground Beef and Avocado (p.33)	Fresh Berry Almond Flour Tart (p.53)	Warm Steak Salad with Arugula, Walnuts, and Blue Cheese (p.61)
Day 14	Savory Turkey Breakfast Meatloaf (p.14)	Grilled Beef Burger with Cheddar and Avocado (p.40)	Sugar-Free Lime Tart (p.51)	Grilled Sardines with Lemon and Herb Oil (p.65)
Day 15	Spinach Waffles with Mustard Sauce and Eggs (p.21)	Spiced Pumpkin & Turmeric Soup (p.30)	Espresso Chocolate Hazelnut Truffles (p.49)	Lemon Herb Chicken Drumsticks with Zucchini Fries (p.68)

Day	Breakfast	Lunch	Snack	Dinner
Day 16	Coconut Lime Keto Sunrise Shake (p.24)	Garlic Butter Steak with Roasted Asparagus (p.37)	Spiced Pumpkin Cheesecake Cups (p.50)	Smoky BBQ Ribs with Roasted Brussels Sprouts (p.69)
Day 17	Ground Beef and Squash Hash with Bell Peppers (p.17)	Spinach and Sausage Shirataki Pasta (p.35)	Zucchini Roll-Ups with Herbed Ricotta (p.43)	Beef and Mushroom Casserole with Almond Flour Crust (p.69)
Day 18	Beef, Spinach, and Cheddar Waffle Sandwich (p.18)	Keto BBQ Pulled Pork with Coleslaw (p.40)	Bacon-Wrapped Green Beans (p.44)	Dill-Crusted Salmon with Cucumber and Feta Salad (p.67)
Day 19	Smoked Salmon Eggs Benedict with Lemon Hollandaise (p.16)	Cheesy Cauliflower Risotto with Mushrooms (p.35)	Sun-Dried Tomato and Walnut Spread (p.45)	Grilled Chicken Salad with Lemon-Parmesan Dressing (p.60)
Day 20	Lentil Crepes with Chicken and Vegetables (p.27)	Herb-Crusted Pork Chops with Zucchini Ribbons (p.36)	Keto Cinnamon Almond Cookies (p.53)	Butter-Poached Lobster with Cauliflower Puree (p.66)
Day 21	Turkey Lettuce Wraps with Mozzarella and Herbs (p.19)	Creamy Chicken Zucchini Noodle Soup (p.28)	Almond Flour Chocolate Chip Brownies (p.51)	Shrimp Scampi with Lemon Garlic Cauliflower Rice (p.65)
Day 22	Quick Cream Cheese Pancakes with Butter (p.22)	Spaghetti Carbonara with Zucchini Noodles (p.34)	Espresso Chocolate Hazelnut Truffles (p.49)	Roasted Eggplant and Bell Pepper Salad with Tahini Dressing (p.63)
Day 23	Green Detox Spinach Smoothie (p.23)	Keto Burrito Bowl with Ground Beef and Avocado (p.33)	Keto Vanilla Coconut Custard (p.49)	BBQ Pork Ribs with Roasted Brussels Sprouts (p.69)
Day 24	Coconut Lime Keto Sunrise Shake (p.24)	Pork & Brussels Sprouts Bowl with Garlic Butter (p.32)	Zucchini Roll-Ups with Herbed Ricotta (p.43)	Beef Tenderloin with Garlic Spinach Cream (p.38)
Day 25	Pesto Mushroom and Bacon Bake (p.15)	Balsamic-Glazed Chicken with Broccoli Mash (p.38)	Keto Mocha Layered Bars (p.50)	Parmesan-Crusted Zucchini Fritters with Lemon Yogurt Sauce (p.56)
Day 26	Egg Crepe Toast with Bacon and Avocado (p.20)	Mushroom and Leek Keto Stew (p.29)	Keto Cinnamon Almond Cookies (p.53)	Vegan Ratatouille with Olives and Basil (p.64)
Day 27	Avocado and Spinach Power Smoothie (p.24)	Garlic Butter Steak with Roasted Asparagus (p.37)	Coconut Raspberry Chia Pudding (p.47)	Seared Steak Bites with Garlic Butter Green Beans (p.58)
Day 28	Family-Style Chorizo Breakfast Bowls (p.25)	Tomato Basil Keto Soup with Parmesan Chips (p.31)	Lemon Garlic Yogurt Dip (p.46)	Mackerel in Lemon Herb Butter with Roasted Asparagus (p.67)
Day 29	Cheddar and Herb Keto Egg Muffins (p.16)	Grilled Chicken with Buttered Asparagus (p.36)	Fresh Berry Almond Flour Tart (p.53)	Beef and Mushroom Casserole with Almond Flour Crust (p.69)
Day 30	Ricotta-Stuffed Peppers with Spinach and Basil (p.18)	Slow-Cooked Turkey and Spinach Stew (p.30)	Sugar-Free Lime Tart (p.51)	Dill-Crusted Salmon with Cucumber and Feta Salad (p.67)

Note: The 30-day meal plan in this book is a flexible guide to help you enjoy a balanced ketogenic diet. Caloric and macronutrient values are approximate and may vary based on ingredients and portion sizes. Adjust portions to suit your dietary needs and health goals. Use this plan as a starting point to explore delicious, nutrient-rich meals while personalizing your keto journey!

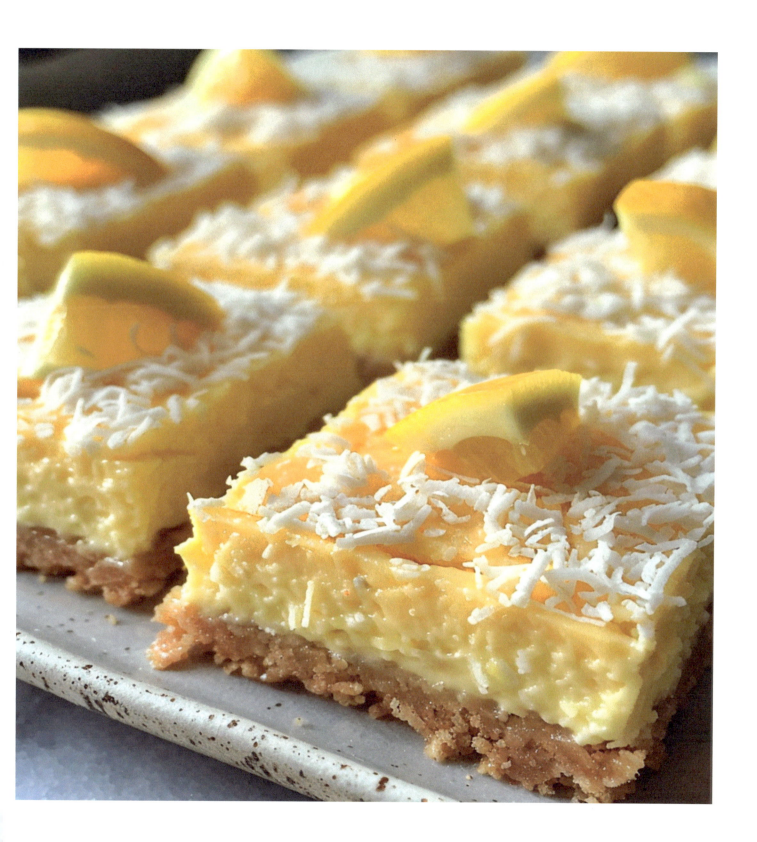

CHAPTER 3: BREAKFASTS: Wholesome & Satisfying Keto Mornings

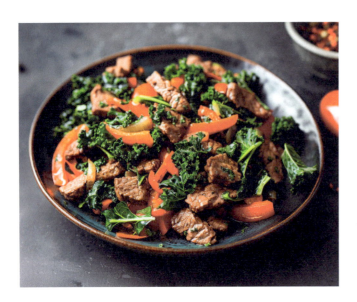

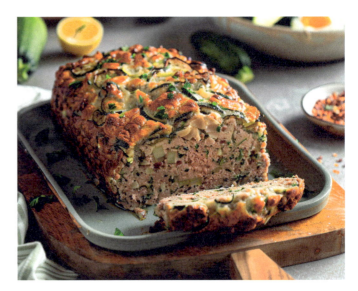

Beef and Kale Power Stir-Fry

Prep: 10 minutes | Cook: 15 minutes | Serves: 1

Ingredients:

- 6 oz lean ground beef (170g)
- 2 cups chopped kale (100g)
- 1/2 cup diced bell peppers (75g)
- 1/4 cup chopped onion (40g)
- 1 tbsp olive oil (15ml)
- 1 tsp minced garlic (5g)
- 1 tsp soy sauce (5ml)
- 1/2 tsp smoked paprika
- Salt and pepper to taste

Instructions:

1. Heat olive oil in a skillet over medium heat. Add ground beef and cook until browned, breaking apart with a spoon.
2. Add onions, garlic, and bell peppers. Cook for 3–4 minutes, stirring occasionally, until softened.
3. Toss in kale, soy sauce, smoked paprika, salt, and pepper. Stir-fry for 2–3 minutes, until kale is wilted and tender.

Nutritional Facts (Per Serving): Calories: 748 | Carbs: 11g | Protein: 24g | Fat: 16g | Fiber: 7g | Sodium: 780mg | Sugars: 9g

Savory Turkey Breakfast Meatloaf

Prep: 10 minutes | Cook: 40 minutes | Serves: 1

Ingredients:

- 6 oz ground turkey (170 g)
- 1/4 cup almond flour (30 g)
- 1/4 cup grated Parmesan cheese (25 g)
- 1/2 cup shredded zucchini (60 g)
- 1/4 cup diced onion (40 g)
- 1 tsp low-carb sweetener
- 1 large egg
- 1/2 tsp garlic powder
- 1/2 tsp onion powder
- 1/4 tsp black pepper
- 1/2 tsp salt
- 1 tbsp olive oil (15 ml)

Instructions:

1. Preheat oven to 375°F (190°C) and grease a small loaf pan with 1 tbsp olive oil.
2. In a bowl, mix ground turkey, egg, almond flour, Parmesan, zucchini, onion, sweetener, and spices. Press evenly into the loaf pan.
3. Bake for 35–40 minutes until fully cooked.

Nutritional Facts (Per Serving): Calories: 750 | Carbs: 10g | Protein: 25g | Fat: 15g | Fiber: 6g | Sodium: 800mg | Sugars: 7g

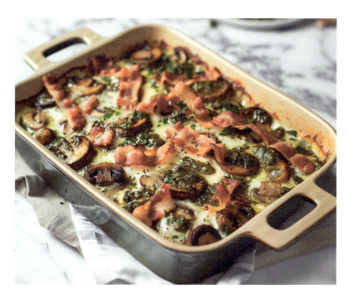

Pesto Mushroom and Bacon Bake

Prep: 10 minutes | Cook: 30 minutes | Serves: 1

Ingredients:

- 3 strips bacon, cooked and crumbled (45g)
- 1 1/2 cups mushrooms, sliced (100g)
- 1/3 cup shredded mozzarella cheese (35g)
- 1 large egg
- 2 tbsp basil pesto (30g)
- 2 tbsp heavy cream (30ml)
- 1 tsp olive oil (5ml)
- 1/4 tsp garlic powder
- Salt and pepper to taste

Instructions:

1. Preheat oven to 375°F (190°C) and grease a small baking dish with olive oil.
2. In a skillet, sauté mushrooms with olive oil and garlic powder over medium heat for 5–7 minutes, or until fully softened.
3. In a bowl, whisk together eggs, heavy cream, pesto, salt, and pepper.
4. Layer cooked mushrooms and crumbled bacon in the baking dish, then pour the egg mixture over. Sprinkle mozzarella cheese evenly on top.
5. Bake for 25–30 minutes, or until eggs are set and cheese is golden.

Nutritional Facts (Per Serving): Calories: 748 | Carbs: 9g | Protein: 31g | Fat: 60g | Fiber: 2g | Sodium: 850mg | Sugars: 2g

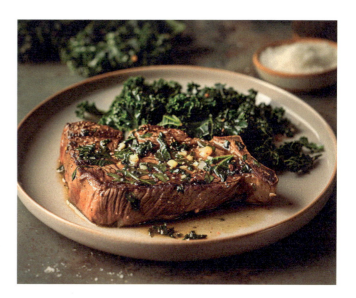

Garlic Butter Steak with Crispy Kale Chips

Prep: 10 minutes | Cook: 20 minutes | Serves: 1

Ingredients:

- 6 oz ribeye steak (170g)
- 2 cups kale leaves, de-stemmed (100g)
- 2 tbsp butter (30g)
- 1 tbsp olive oil (15ml)
- 2 cloves garlic, minced (10g)
- 1/2 tsp smoked paprika
- 1/4 tsp salt
- 1/4 tsp black pepper

Instructions:

1. Preheat the oven to 375°F (190°C).
Toss kale with olive oil and salt, spread on a baking sheet, and bake for 10–12 minutes, flipping once, until crispy.
2. Season the steak (1-inch thick) with salt, pepper, and paprika. Heat a skillet, melt 1 tbsp butter, and sear the steak for 3–4 minutes per side.
3. Let rest for 5 minutes. Add remaining butter and garlic to the skillet, cook for 30 seconds, then slice the steak, drizzle with garlic butter, and serve with kale chips.

Nutritional Facts (Per Serving): Calories: 752 | Carbs: 9g | Protein: 25g | Fat: 16g | Fiber: 5g | Sodium: 780mg | Sugars: 7g

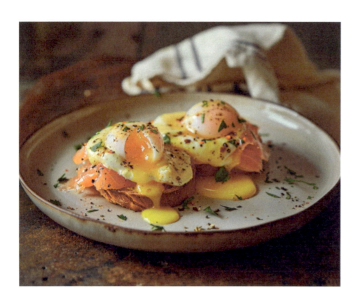

Smoked Salmon Eggs Benedict with Lemon Hollandaise

Prep: 10 minutes | Cook: 20 minutes | Serves: 1

Ingredients:

- 2 large eggs
- 1 English muffin, halved (60g)
- 2 oz smoked salmon (60g)
- 1/4 cup unsalted butter (60g)
- 1 egg yolk
- 1 tbsp lemon juice (15ml)
- 1/4 tsp salt (1.5g)
- 1/8 tsp cayenne pepper (optional)

Instructions:

1. Poach the eggs in simmering water for 3-4 minutes, then remove and set aside.
2. Toast the English muffin halves until golden.
3. In a heatproof bowl, whisk the egg yolk, lemon juice, and salt. Place the bowl over a saucepan of simmering water and whisk continuously while gradually adding melted butter. Whisk until the mixture thickens to a hollandaise consistency.
4. Place smoked salmon on each muffin half, top with a poached egg, and drizzle with the lemon hollandaise. Sprinkle with cayenne if desired.

Nutritional Facts (Per Serving): Calories: 751 | Carbs: 26g | Protein: 24g | Fat: 47g | Fiber: 5g | Sodium: 790mg | Sugars: 7g

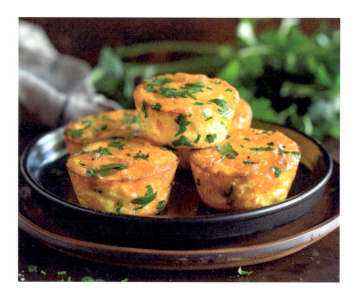

Cheddar and Herb Keto Egg Muffins

Prep: 10 minutes | Cook: 25 minutes | Serves: 1

Ingredients:

- 4 large eggs
- 1/4 cup heavy cream (60ml)
- 1/2 cup shredded cheddar cheese (50g)
- 1/4 tsp black pepper (1.5g)
- 1/4 cup chopped fresh herbs (e.g., parsley,chives) (10g)
- 1/4 tsp salt (1.5g)
- 1 tbsp olive oil (15 ml)

Instructions:

1. Preheat the oven to 350°F (175°C) and grease a muffin tin with olive oil.
2. In a mixing bowl, whisk together eggs, cream, salt, and pepper. Stir in the cheddar cheese and herbs.
3. Pour the egg mixture evenly into 4 muffin cups, filling each about 3/4 full.
4. Bake for 20–25 minutes, or until set and golden on top.
5. Let the muffins cool in the tin for 5 minutes before carefully removing and serving.

Nutritional Facts (Per Serving): Calories: 508 | Carbs: 3g | Protein: 33g | Fat: 40g | Fiber: 0g | Sodium: 660mg | Sugars: 1g

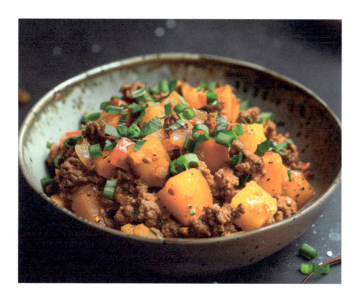

Ground Beef and Squash Hash with Bell Peppers

Prep: 10 minutes | Cook: 20 minutes | Serves: 1

Ingredients:

- 6 oz ground beef (170g)
- 1 cup diced yellow squash (130g)
- 1/2 cup diced red bell pepper (75g)
- 1/4 cup diced onion (40g)
- 1 tbsp olive oil (15 ml)
- 1/2 tsp garlic powder (2g)
- 1/2 tsp smoked paprika (2g)
- 1/4 tsp salt (1.5g)
- 1/4 tsp black pepper (1.5g)

Instructions:

1. Heat olive oil in a skillet over medium heat. Add ground beef and cook until browned, breaking it apart with a spoon. If necessary, drain excess fat.
2. In the same skillet, sauté onion, squash, and bell pepper for 5–7 minutes, or until softened.
3. Return the beef to the skillet and season with garlic powder, smoked paprika, salt, and pepper. Stir and cook for an additional 3–4 minutes.
4. Serve hot, garnished with fresh parsley or avocado slices if desired.

Nutritional Facts (Per Serving): Calories: 540 | Carbs: 9g | Protein: 36g | Fat: 36g | Fiber: 3g | Sodium: 560mg | Sugars: 6g

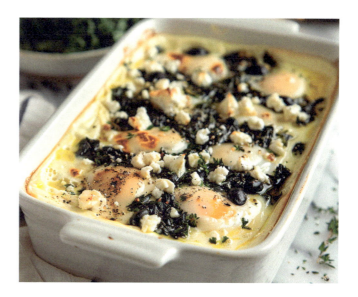

Greek Egg Bake with Feta, Spinach, and Olives

Prep: 10 minutes | Cook: 30 minutes | Serves: 1

Ingredients:

- 4 large eggs
- 1/4 cup heavy cream (60 ml)
- 1/2 cup chopped fresh spinach (20g)
- 1/4 cup crumbled feta cheese (50g)
- 2 tbsp chopped Kalamata olives (20g)
- 1/4 tsp dried oregano (1g)
- 1/4 tsp salt (1.5g)
- 1 tbsp olive oil (15 ml)

Instructions:

1. Preheat the oven to 375°F (190°C) and grease a small baking dish with olive oil.
2. Squeeze chopped spinach with paper towels or a clean kitchen cloth to remove excess moisture.
3. In a mixing bowl, whisk together eggs, cream, salt, and oregano. Stir in spinach, feta, and olives.
4. Pour the mixture into the prepared baking dish and bake for 25–30 minutes, or until set and golden.

Nutritional Facts (Per Serving): Calories: 560 | Carbs: 6g | Protein: 28g | Fat: 45g | Fiber: 2g | Sodium: 690mg | Sugars: 4g

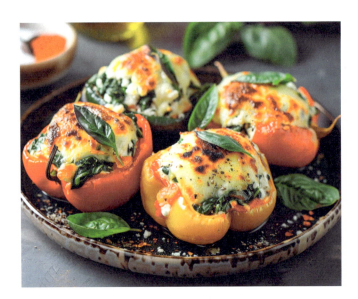

Ricotta-Stuffed Peppers with Spinach and Basil

Prep: 10 minutes | Cook: 25 minutes | Serves: 1

Ingredients:

- 2 medium red bell peppers, halved and deseeded (250g)
- 1/2 cup ricotta cheese (125g)
- 1/2 cup fresh spinach, chopped (20g)
- 1/4 cup grated Parmesan cheese (25g)
- 1 tbsp fresh basil, chopped (5g)
- 1/4 tsp garlic powder (1g)
- 1/4 tsp salt (1.5g)
- 1/4 tsp black pepper (1.5g)
- 1 tbsp olive oil (15 ml)

Instructions:

1. Preheat the oven to 375°F (190°C).
2. In a bowl, mix ricotta, spinach, Parmesan, basil, garlic powder, salt, and black pepper. Fill bell pepper halves, drizzle with olive oil, and bake for 20-25 minutes until tender and golden.

Nutritional Facts (Per Serving): Calories: 520 | Carbs: 10g | Protein: 21g | Fat: 42g | Fiber: 4g | Sodium: 650mg | Sugars: 6g

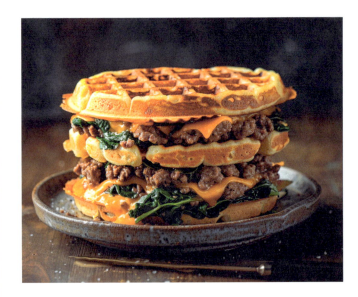

Beef, Spinach, and Cheddar Waffle Sandwich

Prep: 10 minutes | Cook: 15 minutes | Serves: 1

Ingredients:

- 6 oz ground beef (170g)
- 1/2 cup fresh spinach, chopped (20g)
- 1/2 cup shredded cheddar cheese (50g)
- 1 large egg
- 1 tbsp almond flour (7g)
- 1/4 tsp salt (1.5g)
- 1/4 tsp black pepper (1.5g)
- 1 tbsp butter (15g)

Instructions:

1. Cook ground beef in a skillet with salt and pepper until browned; set aside. Whisk egg and almond flour, then mix in cheddar and spinach.
2. Preheat and grease a waffle iron, cook the mixture for 3-5 minutes until golden. Assemble the sandwich with beef between waffle halves.

Nutritional Facts (Per Serving): Calories: 540 | Carbs: 7g | Protein: 27g | Fat: 42g | Fiber: 3g | Sodium: 670mg | Sugars: 5g

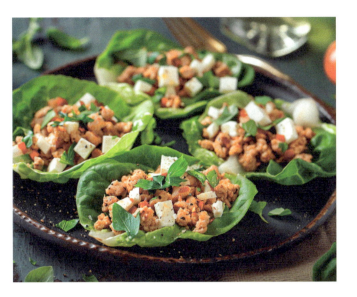

Turkey Lettuce Wraps with Mozzarella and Herbs

Prep: 10 minutes | Cook: 10 minutes | Serves: 1

Ingredients:

- 6 oz ground turkey (170g)
- 4 large lettuce leaves (100g)
- 1/2 cup shredded mozzarella cheese (50g)
- 1/4 cup fresh parsley, chopped (10g)
- 1 tbsp olive oil (15ml)
- 1/4 tsp garlic powder (1g)
- 1/4 tsp salt (1.5g)
- 1/4 tsp black pepper (1.5g)

Instructions:

1. Heat olive oil in a skillet over medium heat. Add ground turkey, breaking it apart with a spoon, and cook for 5–7 minutes, or until fully browned. Season with garlic powder, salt, and black pepper.
2. Pat the lettuce leaves dry with a paper towel and lay them flat on a plate.
3. Evenly divide the cooked turkey among the lettuce leaves.
4. Top each wrap with shredded mozzarella and sprinkle with chopped parsley.

Nutritional Facts (Per Serving): Calories: 475 | Carbs: 5g | Protein: 36g | Fat: 34g | Fiber: 2g | Sodium: 650mg | Sugars: 3g

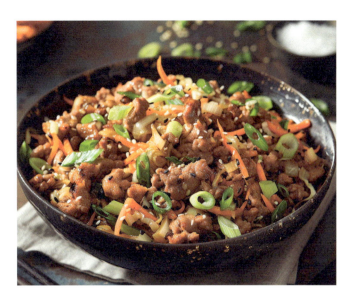

Pork Egg Roll Bowl with Ginger and Scallions

Prep: 10 minutes | Cook: 15 minutes | Serves: 1

Ingredients:

- 6 oz ground pork (170g)
- 1 cup shredded cabbage (85g)
- 1/4 cup shredded carrots (30g)
- 1/4 cup sliced scallions (20g)
- 1 tbsp soy sauce or tamari (15ml)
- 1 tsp fresh ginger, grated (5g)
- 1 tbsp sesame oil (15ml)
- 1/4 tsp garlic powder (1g)
- 1/4 tsp salt (1.5g)
- 1/4 tsp black pepper (1.5g

Instructions:

1. Heat sesame oil in a large skillet over medium heat. Add the ground pork and cook for 5–7 minutes, breaking it up with a spoon, until browned and fully cooked.
2. Stir in the shredded cabbage and carrots. Cook for 3–5 minutes, or until the vegetables are tender.
3. Add soy sauce, grated ginger, garlic powder, salt, and black pepper. Stir well to coat the pork and vegetables in the sauce.

Nutritional Facts (Per Serving): Calories: 525 | Carbs: 7g | Protein: 28g | Fat: 41g | Fiber: 3g | Sodium: 650mg | Sugars: 4g

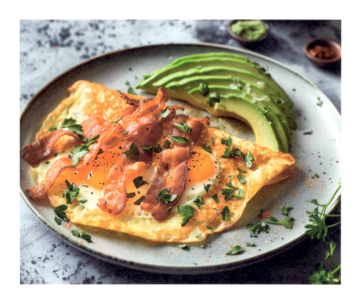

Egg Crepe Toast with Bacon and Avocado

Prep: 10 minutes | Cook: 15 minutes | Serves: 1

Ingredients:

- 3 large eggs
- 1 tbsp heavy cream (15ml)
- 2 slices cooked bacon (30g)
- 1/4 cup shredded cheddar cheese (25g)
- 1 tbsp butter (15g)
- 1/4 tsp salt (1.5g)
- 1/2 avocado, sliced (75g)
- 1/4 tsp black pepper (1.5g)

Instructions:

1. Whisk the eggs, heavy cream, salt, and pepper in a bowl until fully combined.
2. Heat a nonstick skillet over medium heat and melt the butter. Pour in the egg mixture, tilting the skillet to spread it thinly, like a crepe. Cook for 2–3 minutes until set. Adjust heat if necessary for even cooking.
3. Sprinkle shredded cheddar cheese over the crepe and cook for 1 more minute until the cheese melts.
4. Transfer the crepe to a plate, top with bacon and avocado, then fold or roll it up.

Nutritional Facts (Per Serving): Calories: 747 | Carbs: 8g | Protein: 22g | Fat: 64g | Fiber: 6g | Sodium: 780mg | Sugars: 7g

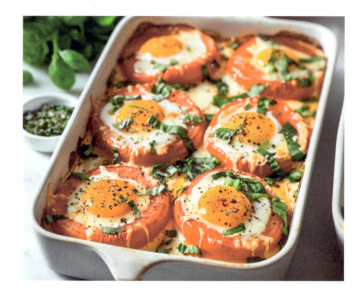

Tomato and Egg Cheese Boats

Prep: 10 minutes | Cook: 20 minutes | Serves: 1

Ingredients:

- 2 large beefsteak tomatoes, halved and cored (400g)
- 1/4 cup shredded mozzarella cheese (25g)
- 1 tbsp grated Parmesan cheese (10g)
- 1 tbsp chopped fresh basil (5g)
- 1/4 tsp garlic powder (1g)
- 1/4 tsp salt (1.5g)
- 2 large eggs
- 1/4 tsp black pepper (1.5g)

Instructions:

1. Preheat the oven to 375°F (190°C) and line a baking dish with parchment paper.
2. Halve and core the tomatoes, then drain them upside down on a paper towel for 5 minutes to remove excess moisture. Place the tomatoes in the baking dish, cut side up.
3. Season the tomatoes with garlic powder, salt, and black pepper. Crack an egg into each tomato half carefully to avoid spilling.
4. Top with mozzarella and Parmesan.
5. Bake for 18–20 minutes, or until the eggs are set to your liking and the cheese is golden.

Nutritional Facts (Per Serving): Calories: 750 | Carbs: 10g | Protein: 20g | Fat: 62g | Fiber: 5g | Sodium: 770mg | Sugars: 8g

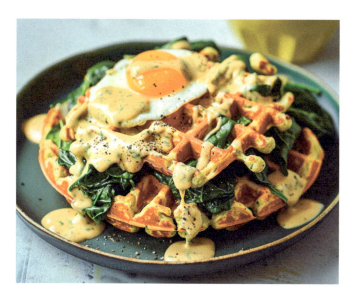

Spinach Waffles with Mustard Sauce and Eggs

Prep: 10 minutes | Cook: 15 minutes | Serves: 1

Ingredients:

- 1/2 cup fresh spinach, finely chopped (20g)
- 2 large eggs
- 1/4 cup almond flour (30g)
- 1/4 cup shredded cheddar cheese (25g)
- 1/2 tsp baking powder (2g)
- 1/4 tsp salt (1.5g)
- 1 tbsp butter, melted (15g)
- 1 tbsp Dijon mustard (15ml)
- 1 tbsp heavy cream (15ml)

Instructions:

1. Preheat and grease a waffle iron. Squeeze moisture from spinach with a paper towel.
2. Mix eggs, almond flour, baking powder, salt, and melted butter in a bowl. Stir in spinach and cheddar.
3. Pour the batter into the preheated waffle iron and cook for 3–5 minutes, or until the waffles are golden and crisp.
4. Whisk Dijon and cream for a sauce and serve with waffles.

Nutritional Facts (Per Serving): Calories: 748 | Carbs: 10g | Protein: 21g | Fat: 62g | Fiber: 6g | Sodium: 780mg | Sugars: 7g

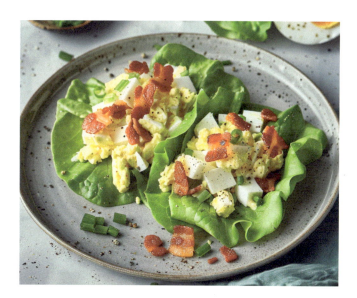

Egg Salad and Bacon Lettuce Cups

Prep: 10 minutes | Cook: 10 minutes | Serves: 1

Ingredients:

- 2 large hard-boiled eggs, chopped
- 2 slices cooked bacon, crumbled (30g)
- 1/4 tsp salt (1.5g)
- 1/4 cup Greek yogurt (60ml)
- 1/4 tsp Dijon mustard (1g)
- 1/4 tsp black pepper (1.5g)
- 4 large lettuce leaves (100g)
- 1 tbsp chopped chives (5g)

Instructions:

1. Boil eggs for 9–10 minutes, cool under cold water, peel, and chop.
2. Mix eggs with bacon, mayo, Dijon, salt, and pepper. Stir until all ingredients are well mixed and the egg salad is creamy. Chill for 10–15 minutes.
3. Arrange lettuce leaves on a serving plate, creating small "cups" with each leaf.
4. Spoon the chilled egg salad evenly into the lettuce cups, filling each one generously. Garnish with chopped chives if desired.

Nutritional Facts (Per Serving): Calories: 753 | Carbs: 7g | Protein: 22g | Fat: 64g | Fiber: 6g | Sodium: 780mg | Sugars: 7g

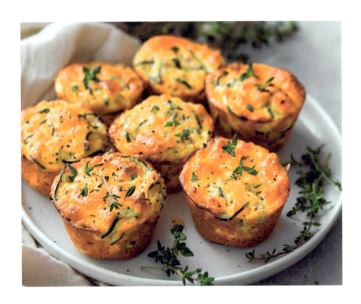

Zucchini and Cheddar Herb Muffins with Thyme

Prep: 10 minutes | Cook: 25 minutes | Serves: 1

Ingredients:

- 1 cup grated zucchini, squeezed to remove excess moisture (150g)
- 2 large eggs
- 1/2 cup almond flour (50g)
- 1/4 cup shredded cheddar cheese (25g)
- 1 tsp fresh thyme leaves (1g)
- 1/2 tsp baking powder (2g)
- 1/4 tsp salt (1.5g)
- 1/4 tsp black pepper (1.5g)
- 1 tbsp olive oil (15ml)

Instructions:

1. Preheat oven to 375°F (190°C) and prepare a muffin tin.
2. Squeeze moisture from grated zucchini using a kitchen towel.
3. Whisk eggs, olive oil, salt, and pepper, then mix in almond flour, baking powder, zucchini, cheese, and thyme.
4. Fill 4 muffin cups 3/4 full and bake for 20–25 minutes until golden and set.

Nutritional Facts (Per Serving): Calories: 750 | Carbs: 11g | Protein: 21g | Fat: 62g | Fiber: 7g | Sodium: 780mg | Sugars: 7g

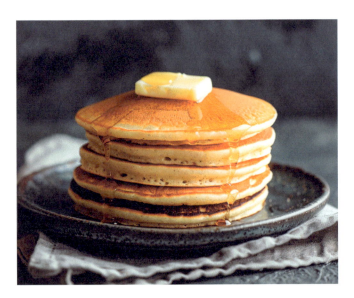

Quick Cream Cheese Pancakes with Butter

Prep: 5 minutes | Cook: 10 minutes | Serves: 1

Ingredients:

- 2 oz cream cheese, softened (60g)
- 2 large eggs
- 1/4 tsp vanilla extract (1ml)
- 1 tbsp almond flour (7g)
- 1/4 tsp baking powder (1g)
- 1 tbsp butter, for cooking (15g)
- 1 tbsp butter, for topping (15g)

Instructions:

1. In a blender or mixing bowl, blend together the cream cheese, eggs, vanilla extract, almond flour, and baking powder until smooth. Ensure no lumps remain for a consistent batter.
2. Heat a nonstick skillet over medium heat and melt 1 tbsp of butter for cooking.
3. Pour small amounts of batter (about 2 tbsp per pancake) onto the skillet, cooking 2–3 pancakes at a time. Cook for 1–2 minutes on each side, or until golden brown.
4. Stack the pancakes on a plate and top with the remaining butter.

Nutritional Facts (Per Serving): Calories: 749 | Carbs: 8g | Protein: 22g | Fat: 64g | Fiber: 5g | Sodium: 760mg | Sugars: 7g

CHAPTER 5: BREAKFASTS: Power-Packed Keto Smoothies & Shakes

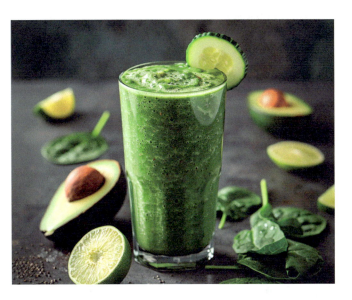

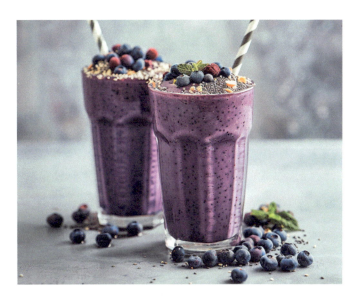

Green Detox Spinach Smoothie

Prep: 5 minutes | Cook: 1 minutes | Serves: 1

Ingredients:

- 1 cup fresh spinach (30g)
- 1/2 avocado, peeled and pitted (75g)
- 1/2 cup unsweetened almond milk (120 ml)
- 1/4 cup Greek yogurt (60g)
- 1/2 cucumber, chopped (75g)
- 1 tbsp lime juice (15 ml)
- 1/2 tsp low carb sweetener (2g)
- 3-4 ice cubes

Instructions:

1. Add the spinach, avocado, almond milk, Greek yogurt, cucumber, lime juice, and low-carb sweetener to a blender.
2. Blend on high speed until smooth and creamy.
3. Add the ice cubes and blend again until the smoothie reaches your desired texture.
4. Pour into a glass and serve immediately.

Nutritional Facts (Per Serving): Calories: 742 | Carbs: 12g | Protein: 20g | Fat: 61g | Fiber: 8g | Sodium: 780mg | Sugars: 7g

Blueberry Antioxidant Shake

Prep: 5 minutes | Cook: 1 minutes | Serves: 1

Ingredients:

- 1/2 cup fresh or frozen blueberries (75g)
- 1 cup unsweetened almond milk (240 ml)
- 1/4 cup Greek yogurt (60g)
- 1 tbsp almond butter (15g)
- 1/2 tsp low carb sweetener (2g)
- 1/2 tsp vanilla extract (2 ml)
- 3-4 ice cubes

Instructions:

1. Place the blueberries (fresh or frozen), almond milk, Greek yogurt, almond butter, low-carb sweetener, and vanilla extract in a blender.
2. Blend on high until smooth and creamy. For a thicker shake, use frozen blueberries.
3. Add the ice cubes and blend again to thicken and chill the shake.

Nutritional Facts (Per Serving): Calories: 747 | Carbs: 15g | Protein: 19g | Fat: 58g | Fiber: 6g | Sodium: 760mg | Sugars: 10g

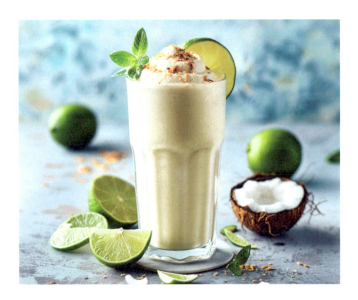

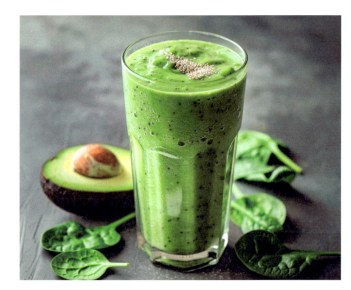

Coconut Lime Keto Sunrise Shake

Prep: 5 minutes | Cook: 1 minutes | Serves: 1

Ingredients:

- 1/2 cup unsweetened coconut milk (120 ml)
- 1/4 cup full-fat coconut cream (60g)
- 2 tbsp fresh lime juice (30ml)
- 1 tbsp low carb sweetener (12g)
- 1 scoop vanilla protein powder (30g)
- 1/4 tsp lime zest (1g)
- 3-4 ice cubes

Instructions:

1. Chill the coconut milk and cream in the refrigerator for at least 1 hour before blending.
2. Add coconut milk, coconut cream, lime juice, low-carb sweetener, vanilla protein powder, and lime zest to a blender.
3. Blend on high until smooth and creamy.
4. Add ice cubes and blend again to chill the shake. Pour into a glass, garnish with additional lime zest if desired, and serve immediately.

Nutritional Facts (Per Serving): Calories: 751 | Carbs: 10g | Protein: 20g | Fat: 64g | Fiber: 7g | Sodium: 760mg | Sugars: 8g

Avocado and Spinach Power Smoothie

Prep: 5 minutes | Cook: 1 minutes | Serves: 1

Ingredients:

- 1 cup fresh spinach (30g)
- 1/2 avocado, peeled and pitted (75g)
- 1/2 cup unsweetened almond milk (120 ml)
- 1 scoop plain or vanilla protein powder (30g)
- 1/4 cup Greek yogurt (60g)
- 1 tbsp low carb sweetener (12g)
- 1 tbsp fresh lemon juice (15ml)
- 3-4 ice cubes

Instructions:

1. Add spinach, avocado, almond milk, Greek yogurt, protein powder, low carb sweetener, and lemon juice to a blender.
2. Blend on high until the mixture is smooth and creamy.
3. Add ice cubes and blend again to achieve a chilled texture.
4. Pour into a glass and serve immediately.

Nutritional Facts (Per Serving): Calories: 749 | Carbs: 11g | Protein: 24g | Fat: 60g | Fiber: 8g | Sodium: 780mg | Sugars: 9g

CHAPTER 6: BREAKFASTS: Family-Friendly Keto Brunch Ideas

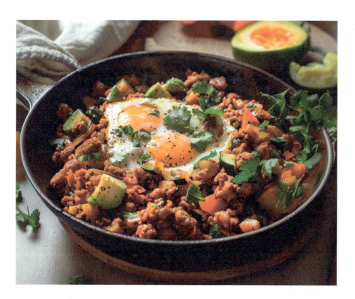

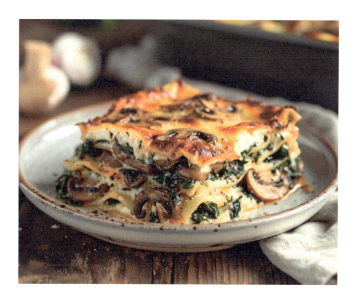

Family-Style Chorizo Breakfast Bowls

Prep: 10 minutes | Cook: 20 minutes | Serves: 1

Ingredients:

- 4 oz ground chorizo sausage (120g)
- 1/2 cup diced bell peppers (75g)
- 1/2 cup diced zucchini (75g)
- 1/4 cup shredded cheddar cheese (25g)
- 1 tbsp olive oil (15ml)
- 1/4 tsp garlic powder (1g)
- 1/4 tsp paprika (1g)
- 1/4 tsp salt (1.5g)
- 2 large eggs
- 1/4 tsp black pepper (1.5g)

Instructions:

1. Heat olive oil in a skillet over medium heat. Cook chorizo for 5-7 minutes until browned.
2. Add bell peppers, zucchini, and seasonings; sauté for 5 minutes. Push to one side, cook eggs on the other for 3-4 minutes.

Nutritional Facts (Per Serving): Calories: 750 | Carbs: 12g | Protein: 23g | Fat: 61g | Fiber: 7g | Sodium: 780mg | Sugars: 8g

Spinach and Mushroom Keto Lasagna

Prep: 15 minutes | Cook: 40 minutes | Serves: 1

Ingredients:

- 1/2 tsp Italian seasoning (2g)
- 1 cup mushrooms, sliced (90g)
- 1 cup ricotta cheese (250g)
- 1 cup shredded mozzarella cheese (100g)
- 1/4 cup grated Parmesan cheese (25g)
- 1/2 cup marinara sauce, no sugar added (120ml)
- 1 large egg
- 1 tbsp olive oil (15ml)
- 1 cup fresh spinach,(30g)
- 1/4 tsp garlic powder(1g)
- 1/4 tsp salt (1.5g)

Instructions:

1. Preheat oven to 375°F (190°C) and grease a dish. Sauté mushrooms, spinach, garlic, and salt. Mix ricotta, egg, Parmesan, and seasoning.
2. Layer marinara, ricotta, veggies, and mozzarella. Bake 35-40 minutes until golden.

Nutritional Facts (Per Serving): Calories: 748 | Carbs: 14g | Protein: 22g | Fat: 62g | Fiber: 6g | Sodium: 790mg | Sugars: 9g

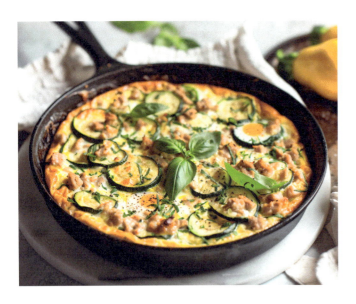

Turkey and Zucchini Breakfast Frittata

Prep: 10 minutes | Cook: 25 minutes | Serves: 1

Ingredients:

- 4 oz ground turkey (120g)
- 1/2 cup grated zucchini, squeezed to remove moisture (75g)
- 4 large eggs
- 1/4 cup heavy cream (60ml)
- 1/2 cup shredded mozzarella cheese (50g)
- 1 tbsp olive oil (15 ml)
- 1/4 tsp garlic powder (1g)
- 1/4 tsp salt (1.5g)
- 1/4 tsp black pepper (1.5g)

Instructions:

1. Preheat oven to 375°F (190°C) and grease a baking dish.
2. Cook turkey in olive oil for 5-7 minutes. Add grated zucchini (squeezed to remove excess moisture), garlic powder, salt, and pepper.
3. Whisk eggs, cream, and mozzarella. Spread turkey and zucchini in the dish, pour egg mixture over.
4. Bake 20-25 minutes until set and golden.

Nutritional Facts (Per Serving): Calories: 749 | Carbs: 10g | Protein: 24g | Fat: 61g | Fiber: 6g | Sodium: 770mg | Sugars: 7g

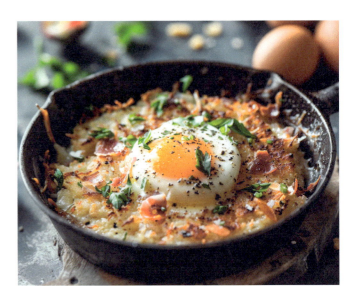

Almond Flour Hash Browns with Sour Cream

Prep: 10 minutes | Cook: 20 minutes | Serves: 1

Ingredients:

- 1/2 cup almond flour (50g)
- 1/4 cup grated Parmesan cheese (25g)
- 1 large egg
- 2 tbsp unsalted butter, melted (30g)
- 1/4 tsp garlic powder (1g)
- 1/4 tsp salt (1.5g)
- 1/4 tsp black pepper (1.5g)
- 1/4 cup sour cream, for topping (60g)

Instructions:

1. In a mixing bowl, combine almond flour, Parmesan cheese, garlic powder, salt, and black pepper. Stir in the egg and melted butter until the mixture forms a dough-like consistency.
2. Shape the mixture into small patties, about 2-3 inches in diameter.
3. Heat a nonstick skillet over medium heat and add a little butter or oil. Cook the patties for 3-4 minutes per side, or until golden brown and crispy.

Nutritional Facts (Per Serving): Calories: 750 | Carbs: 8g | Protein: 19g | Fat: 63g | Fiber: 7g | Sodium: 780mg | Sugars: 7g

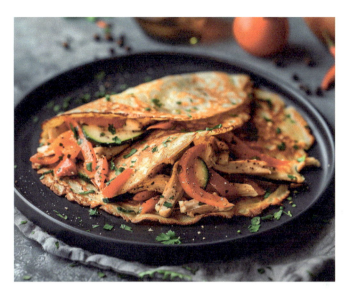

Lentil Crepes with Chicken and Vegetables

Prep: 15 minutes | Cook: 20 minutes | Serves: 1

Ingredients:

- 1/4 cup almond flour (30g)
- 1/4 cup water (60 ml)
- 4 oz cooked chicken breast, shredded (120g)
- 1/2 cup sautéed mixed vegetables (e.g., zucchini, bell peppers, onions) (75g)
- 1/4 cup shredded mozzarella cheese (25g)
- 1/4 tsp garlic powder (1g)
- 1/4 tsp salt (1.5g)
- 1/4 tsp black pepper (1.5g)
- 1 large egg
- 1 tbsp olive oil (15ml)

Instructions:

1. In a bowl, whisk together almond flour, water, egg, and salt until smooth.
2. Heat 1/2 tbsp olive oil in a nonstick skillet over medium heat. Pour in half the batter, tilting the skillet to spread it thinly. Cook for 2-3 minutes on each side until golden. Repeat with the remaining batter to make two crepes.
3. Fill each crepe with shredded chicken, sautéed vegetables, and mozzarella cheese. Sprinkle with garlic powder and black pepper.

Nutritional Facts (Per Serving): Calories: 743 | Carbs: 10g | Protein: 24g | Fat: 60g | Fiber: 6g | Sodium: 780mg | Sugars: 4g

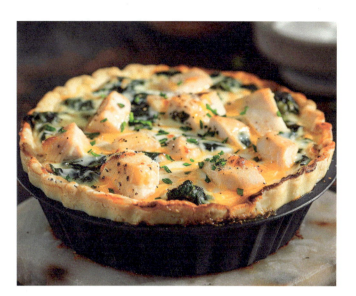

Cheesy Chicken and Spinach Breakfast Quiche

Prep: 10 minutes | Cook: 35 minutes | Serves: 1

Ingredients:

- 4 large eggs
- 1/4 cup heavy cream (60ml)
- 1 cup fresh spinach, chopped (30g)
- 1/2 cup cooked chicken breast, diced (75g)
- 1/2 cup shredded cheddar cheese (50g)
- 1/4 cup grated Parmesan cheese (25g)
- 1 tbsp butter, for greasing (15g)
- 1/4 tsp garlic powder (1g)
- 1/4 tsp salt (1.5g)
- 1/4 tsp black pepper (1.5g)

Instructions:

1. Preheat the oven to 375°F (190°C). Grease a small pie dish or oven-safe skillet with butter.
2. In a mixing bowl, whisk together eggs, heavy cream, garlic powder, salt, and black pepper.
3. Stir in the chopped spinach, diced chicken, and cheddar cheese.
4. Pour the mixture into the prepared dish and sprinkle Parmesan cheese evenly on top.
5. Bake for 30-35 minutes, or until the quiche is set and golden. Let rest for 10 minutes before slicing.

Nutritional Facts (Per Serving): Calories: 750 | Carbs: 10g | Protein: 23g | Fat: 61g | Fiber: 5g | Sodium: 790mg | Sugars: 8g

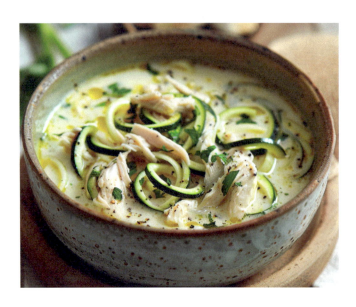

Creamy Chicken Zucchini Noodle Soup

Prep: 15 minutes | Cook: 20 minutes | Serves: 4

Ingredients:

- 2 cups shredded cooked chicken (250g)
- 4 cups chicken broth (1L)
- 1/2 cup coconut cream (120ml)
- 1 tbsp olive oil (15ml)
- 1 small onion, diced (70g)
- 2 garlic cloves, minced (6g)
- 1 tsp Italian seasoning (5g)
- 2 small zucchini, spiralized (200g)
- Salt and pepper to taste

Instructions:

1. Heat olive oil in a large pot over medium heat. Sauté onion and garlic for 3-4 minutes until softened.
2. Add broth, coconut cream, seasoning, salt, and pepper; simmer. Stir in chicken and zucchini noodles, cooking for 2-3 minutes until tender.

Nutritional Facts (Per Serving): Calories: 498 | Carbs: 14g | Protein: 20g | Fat: 16g | Fiber: 5g | Sodium: 450mg | Sugars: 4g

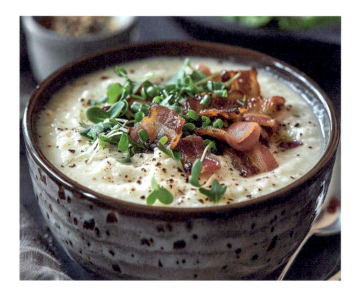

Savory Bacon and Cauliflower Soup

Prep: 10 minutes | Cook: 25 minutes | Serves: 4

Ingredients:

- 4 slices cooked bacon, crumbled (60g)
- 3 1/2 cups cauliflower florets (500g)
- 3 cups chicken broth (750ml)
- 1 cup unsweetened almond milk (240ml)
- 1 small onion, diced (70g)
- 2 garlic cloves, minced (6g)
- 1 tbsp butter (15g)
- 1 tsp smoked
- paprika (5g)
- Salt and pepper to taste
- Fresh parsley or extra bacon bits for garnish (optional)

Instructions:

1. Melt butter in a pot and sauté onion and garlic for 3-4 minutes.Add cauliflower, broth, almond milk, paprika, salt, and pepper; simmer for 15 minutes.
2. Blend until smooth, stir in bacon, and garnish with parsley or bacon bits.

Nutritional Facts (Per Serving): Calories: 500 | Carbs: 18g | Protein: 17g | Fat: 20g | Fiber: 6g | Sodium: 520mg | Sugars: 6g

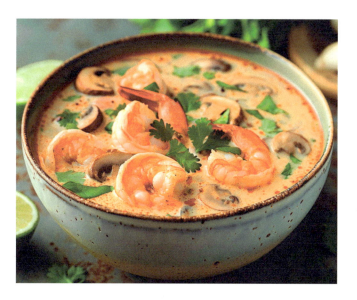

Keto Thai Coconut Shrimp Soup

Prep: 10 minutes | Cook: 20 minutes | Serves: 4

Ingredients:

- 1 lb shrimp, peeled and deveined (450g)
- 4 cups coconut milk (1L)
- 2 cups chicken broth (500ml)
- 2 tbsp red curry paste (30g)
- 1 tbsp fish sauce (15ml)
- 1 tbsp olive oil (15ml)
- 1 red bell pepper, sliced (150g)
- 1 cup mushrooms, sliced (120g)
- 1 small onion, diced (70g)
- 1 tbsp ginger, grated (15g)
- 1 lime, juice and zest
- Fresh cilantro, chopped (for garnish)

Instructions:

1. Heat olive oil in a pot and sauté onion, ginger, and curry paste for 2–3 minutes.
2. Add coconut milk, broth, fish sauce, and lime zest; simmer.
3. Stir in bell peppers, mushrooms, and shrimp, cooking until shrimp are pink and vegetables tender, about 5 minutes.
4. Add lime juice and garnish with cilantro. Adjust spice as desired.

Nutritional Facts (Per Serving): Calories: 503 | Carbs: 26g | Protein: 18g | Fat: 12g | Fiber: 7g | Sodium: 520mg | Sugar: 9g

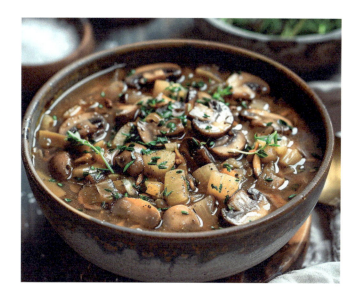

Mushroom and Leek Keto Stew

Prep: 10 minutes | Cook: 25 minutes | Serves: 4

Ingredients:

- 2 cups mushrooms, sliced (300g)
- 2 medium leeks, sliced (150g)
- 3 cups chicken broth (750ml)
- 1 cup heavy cream (240ml)
- 2 garlic cloves, minced (6g)
- 1 tbsp olive oil (15ml)
- 1 tsp thyme (5g)
- Salt and pepper to taste
- Fresh parsley, chopped (for garnish)

Instructions:

1. Heat olive oil in a large pot over medium heat. Sauté garlic and leeks until softened, about 5 minutes.
2. Add the sliced mushrooms and cook for another 5 minutes, stirring occasionally, until the mushrooms release their moisture and begin to brown.
3. Add chicken broth, thyme, salt, and pepper. Simmer for 10 minutes.
4. Stir in heavy cream and simmer for an additional 5 minutes.

Nutritional Facts (Per Serving): Calories: 495 | Carbs: 16g | Protein: 16g | Fat: 11g | Fiber: 6g | Sodium: 500mg | Sugar: 7g

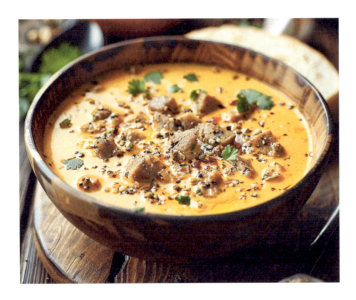

Spiced Pumpkin & Turmeric Soup

Prep: 10 minutes | Cook: 20 minutes | Serves: 4

Ingredients:

- 3 cups pumpkin purée (750g)
- 3 cups vegetable broth (750ml)
- 1 cup coconut milk (240ml)
- 1 small onion, diced (70g)
- 2 garlic cloves, minced (6g)
- 1 tbsp olive oil (15ml)
- 1 tsp ground turmeric (5g)
- 1/2 tsp ground cinnamon (2g)
- Salt and pepper to taste
- Fresh cilantro, chopped (for garnish)

Instructions:

1. Heat olive oil in a large pot over medium heat. Sauté the onion and garlic until softened, about 3-4 minutes.
2. Stir in the turmeric and cinnamon, cooking for 1 minute to release the flavors.
3. Add the unsweetened pumpkin purée, vegetable broth, and coconut milk. Stir well and bring to a gentle simmer.
4. Cook for 10-15 minutes, stirring occasionally. Use an immersion blender to puree the soup until smooth, if desired. Season with salt and pepper; garnish with cilantro.

Nutritional Facts (Per Serving): Calories: 498 | Carbs: 26g | Protein: 14g | Fat: 11g | Fiber: 7g | Sodium: 450mg | Sugar: 8g

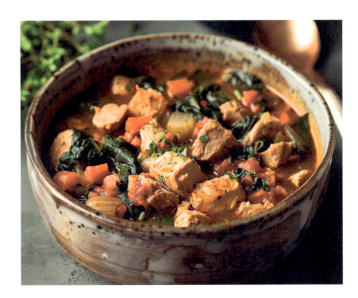

Slow-Cooked Turkey and Spinach Stew

Prep: 15 minutes | Cook: 4 hours | Serves: 4

Ingredients:

- 1 lb turkey breast, diced (450g)
- 4 cups fresh spinach (120g)
- 2 cups chicken broth (500ml)
- 1 cup diced tomatoes (250g)
- 1 small onion, diced (70g)
- 2 garlic cloves
- ,minced (6g)
- 1 tbsp olive oil (15ml)
- 1 tsp dried oregano (5g)
- 1/2 tsp smoked paprika (2g)
- Salt and pepper to taste

Instructions:

1. Heat olive oil in a skillet over medium heat. Sear the turkey pieces until browned on all sides, about 4-5 minutes.
2. Transfer the turkey to a slow cooker. Add fresh spinach (packed), chicken broth, diced tomatoes, onion, garlic, oregano, smoked paprika, salt, and pepper.
3. Stir well, cover, and cook on low for 4 hours, or until the turkey is tender and fully cooked.
4. Serve warm, garnished with optional avocado slices or a dollop of sour cream.

Nutritional Facts (Per Serving): Calories: 496 | Carbs: 22g | Protein: 19g | Fat: 12g | Fiber: 6g | Sodium: 520mg | Sugar: 7g

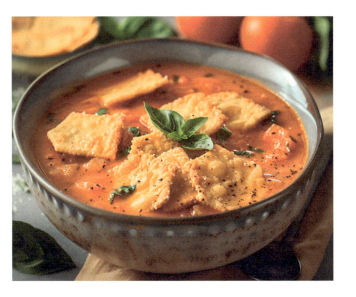

Tomato Basil Keto Soup with Parmesan Chips

Prep: 10 minutes | Cook: 20 minutes | Serves: 4

Ingredients:

- 4 cups diced tomatoes (800g)
- 3 cups chicken broth (750ml)
- 1/2 cup heavy cream (120ml)
- 1 small onion, diced (70g)
- 2 garlic cloves, minced (6g)
- 2 tbsp olive oil (30ml)
- 1 tsp dried basil (5g)
- Salt and pepper to taste
- 1 cup shredded Parmesan cheese (100g)

Instructions:

1. Heat olive oil in a pot over medium heat. Sauté onion and garlic for 3-4 minutes.
2. Add diced tomatoes (no added sugar), broth, basil, salt, and pepper; simmer for 10 minutes.
3. Puree with an immersion blender, stir in cream, and simmer 5 minutes.
4. Preheat the oven to 375°F (190°C). Line a baking sheet with parchment paper. Place tablespoon-sized mounds of Parmesan cheese on the sheet and flatten slightly.
5. Bake for 5-7 minutes, monitoring closely after 5 minutes, until golden and crisp.

Nutritional Facts (Per Serving): Calories: 498 | Carbs: 22g | Protein: 15g | Fat: 12g | Fiber: 7g | Sodium: 530mg | Sugar: 6g

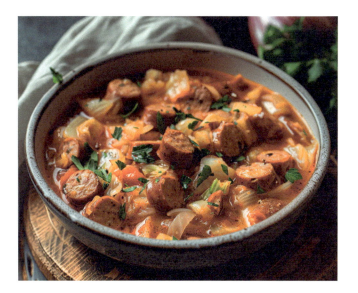

Cabbage and Sausage Soup with Smoked Paprika

Prep: 10 minutes | Cook: 30 minutes | Serves: 4

Ingredients:

- 1 lb smoked sausage, sliced (450g)
- 4 cups shredded cabbage (300g)
- 3 cups chicken broth (750ml)
- 1 cup diced tomatoes (250g)
- 1 small onion, diced (70g)
- 2 garlic cloves, minced (6g)
- 1 tbsp olive oil (15ml)
- 1 tsp smoked paprika (5g)
- Salt and pepper to taste

Instructions:

1. Heat olive oil in a large pot over medium heat. Sauté the onion and garlic until fragrant, about 3 minutes.
2. Add the sliced sausage and cook for 5 minutes until lightly browned.
3. Stir in the cabbage, diced tomatoes, chicken broth, smoked paprika, salt, and pepper. Mix well and bring to a simmer.
4. Cover and cook for 20-25 minutes until the cabbage is tender. Stir occasionally.

Nutritional Facts (Per Serving): Calories: 495 | Carbs: 19g | Protein: 18g | Fat: 13g | Fiber: 6g | Sodium: 520mg | Sugar: 7g

CHAPTER 8: LUNCHES: Creative Keto Bowls & Platters

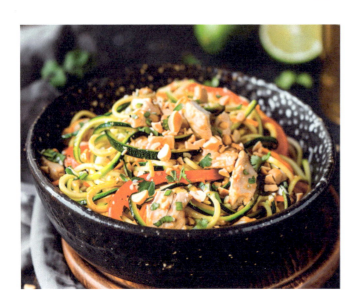

Zucchini Noodle Pad Thai Bowl

Prep: 15 minutes | Cook: 10 minutes | Serves: 4

Ingredients:

- 4 medium zucchini, spiralized (600g)
- 1 lb cooked chicken breast, sliced (450g)
- 2 eggs, whisked
- 2 tbsp soy sauce or tamari (30ml)
- 1 tbsp peanut butter (15g) (unsweetened, natural)
- 1 tbsp sesame oil (15ml)

Instructions:

1. Heat sesame oil in a skillet, scramble eggs until set, and set aside.
2. Cook zucchini noodles for 2 minutes, add chicken, and heat through.
3. Mix soy sauce with unsweetened, natural peanut butter, pour over, and toss.
4. Return eggs, mix, and cook 1 more minute. Garnish with lime or peanuts.

Nutritional Facts (Per Serving): Calories: 500 | Carbs: 18g | Protein: 18g | Fat: 12g | Fiber: 7g | Sodium: 500mg | Sugar: 5g

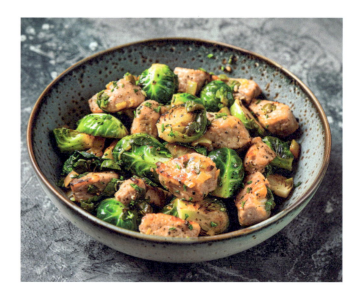

Pork & Brussels Sprouts Bowl with Garlic Butter

Prep: 10 minutes | Cook: 20 minutes | Serves: 4

Ingredients:

- 1 lb ground pork (450g)
- 4 cups Brussels sprouts, halved (500g)
- 3 tbsp butter (45g)
- 2 garlic cloves, minced (6g)
- 1 tsp smoked paprika (5g)
- Salt and pepper to taste

Instructions:

1. Cook ground pork in a skillet for 6-8 minutes until browned, season and set aside. Melt butter in the same skillet, sauté garlic for 1 minute, then add Brussels sprouts and smoked paprika.
2. Cook for 8-10 minutes, stirring occasionally, until tender and caramelized. Return pork to the skillet, mix well, and heat through for 2 minutes.

Nutritional Facts (Per Serving): Calories: 498 | Carbs: 18g | Protein: 19g | Fat: 13g | Fiber: 6g | Sodium: 520mg | Sugar: 7g

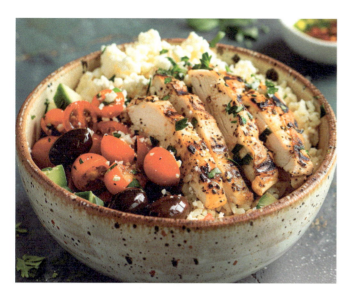

Greek Cauliflower Rice Bowl with Chicken and Feta

Prep: 10 minutes | Cook: 15 minutes | Serves: 4

Ingredients:

- 4 cups riced cauliflower (600g)
- 1 lb cooked chicken breast, diced (450g)
- 1 tsp dried oregano (5g)
- 1/2 cup crumbled feta cheese (100g)
- 1/4 cup Kalamata olives, sliced (60g)
- 2 tbsp olive oil (30ml)
- 1 tbsp lemon juice (15ml)
- 1 cup cherry tomatoes, halved (150g)
- Salt and pepper to taste

Instructions:

1. Heat 1 tbsp olive oil in a skillet over medium heat. Add the riced cauliflower and sauté for 5-7 minutes until tender. Season with salt and pepper.
In a large bowl, combine the cooked cauliflower rice, diced chicken, cherry tomatoes, olives, and feta cheese.
2. In a small bowl, whisk together the remaining olive oil, lemon juice, and oregano. Drizzle over the cauliflower mixture and toss well.

Nutritional Facts (Per Serving): Calories: 494 | Carbs: 18g | Protein: 19g | Fat: 12g | Fiber: 7g | Sodium: 520mg | Sugar: 6g

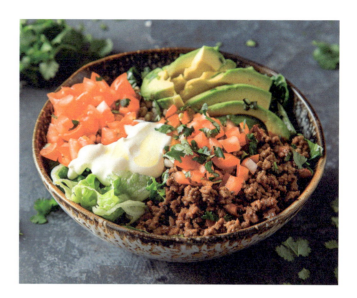

Keto Burrito Bowl with Ground Beef and Avocado

Prep: 10 minutes | Cook: 15 minutes | Serves: 4

Ingredients:

- 1 lb ground beef (450g)
- 4 cups shredded lettuce (200g)
- 1 cup diced tomatoes (250g)
- 1 medium avocado, diced (150g)
- 1/2 cup shredded cheddar cheese (100g)
- 1/4 cup sour cream (60g)
- 2 tsp chili powder (10g)
- 1 tsp ground cumin (5g)
- 1 tbsp olive oil (15ml)
- Salt and pepper to taste

Instructions:

1. Heat olive oil in a skillet over medium heat. Add ground beef, chili powder, cumin, salt, and pepper. Cook for 8-10 minutes, breaking the meat into crumbles, until browned and fully cooked.
2. Divide shredded lettuce evenly into four bowls. Top with cooked ground beef, diced tomatoes, avocado, and shredded cheddar cheese.
3. Add a dollop of sour cream to each bowl.

Nutritional Facts (Per Serving): Calories: 498 | Carbs: 16g | Protein: 18g | Fat: 13g | Fiber: 6g | Sodium: 500mg | Sugar: 5g

CHAPTER 9: LUNCHES: Keto-Friendly Pasta & Risottos

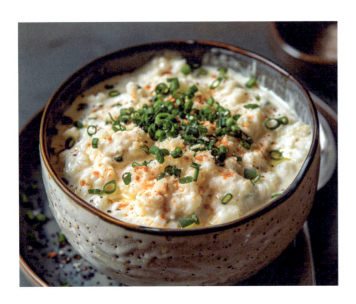

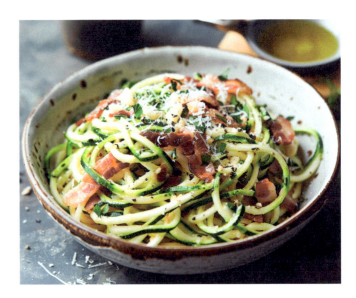

Creamy Garlic Shirataki Alfredo

Prep: 10 minutes | Cook: 15 minutes | Serves: 1

Ingredients:

- 1 package shirataki noodles (200g)
- 1 tbsp butter (14g)
- 1 clove garlic, minced (5g)
- 1/4 cup heavy cream (60ml)
- 1/4 cup grated Parmesan cheese (25g)
- 1/8 tsp ground nutmeg (0.5g)
- Salt and pepper to taste

Instructions:

1. Rinse shirataki noodles under cold water, boil for 2 minutes, then dry in a pan.
2. Melt butter in a skillet, sauté garlic for 1–2 minutes, then add cream, Parmesan, and nutmeg.
3. Add shirataki noodles to the skillet, toss to coat, and heat through. Season with salt and pepper to taste.

Nutritional Facts (Per Serving): Calories: 495 | Carbs: 8g | Protein: 13g | Fat: 12g | Fiber: 7g | Sodium: 550mg | Sugars: 6g

Spaghetti Carbonara with Zucchini Noodles

Prep: 15 minutes | Cook: 10 minutes | Serves: 1

Ingredients:

- 1 medium zucchini, spiralized (200g)
- 2 slices turkey bacon, chopped (50g)
- 1/4 cup grated Parmesan cheese (25g)
- 1 egg, whisked (50g)
- 1/4 tsp garlic powder (1g)
- 1/8 tsp ground black pepper (0.5g)
- 1 tbsp olive oil (14g)

Instructions:

1. Heat olive oil, cook turkey bacon until crispy, and set aside.
2. Sauté zucchini noodles for 2-3 minutes. Off heat, stir in egg,
3. Parmesan, garlic powder, and pepper until coated. Top with bacon and serve warm.

Nutritional Facts (Per Serving): Calories: 493 | Carbs: 10g | Protein: 19g | Fat: 13g | Fiber: 6g | Sodium: 540mg | Sugars: 6g

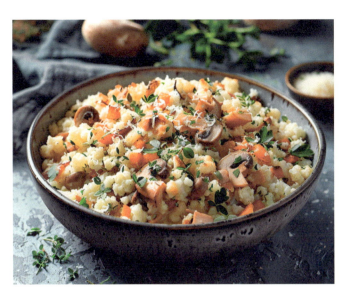

Cheesy Cauliflower Risotto with Mushrooms

Prep: 10 minutes | Cook: 15 minutes | Serves: 1

Ingredients:

- 2 cups cauliflower rice (300g)
- 1 tbsp olive oil (14g)
- 1/2 cup sliced mushrooms (50g)
- 1/4 cup heavy cream (60ml)
- 1/4 cup grated Parmesan cheese (25g)
- 1/4 tsp garlic powder (1g)
- Salt and pepper to taste

Instructions:

1. Heat olive oil in a skillet over medium heat. Sauté mushrooms until tender, about 5 minutes.
2. Add fresh or frozen cauliflower rice to the skillet and cook for 3-4 minutes.
3. Stir in heavy cream, Parmesan cheese, and garlic powder. Cook until creamy, about 2-3 minutes.
4. Season with salt and pepper to taste. Garnish with fresh thyme or parsley before serving.

Nutritional Facts (Per Serving): Calories: 500 | Carbs: 12g | Protein: 15g | Fat: 13g | Fiber: 7g | Sodium: 520mg | Sugars: 7g

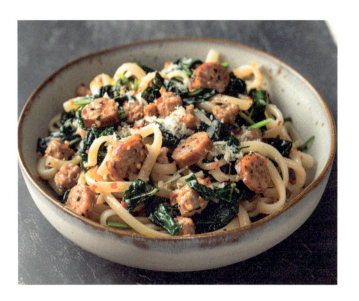

Spinach and Sausage Shirataki Pasta

Prep: 10 minutes | Cook: 10 minutes | Serves: 1

Ingredients:

- 1 package shirataki noodles (200g)
- 2 links turkey sausage, sliced (100g)
- 1 tbsp butter (14g)
- 1 cup fresh spinach (30g)
- 1/4 cup heavy cream (60ml)
- 1/4 cup grated Parmesan cheese (25g)
- 1/4 tsp red pepper flakes (0.5g)
- Salt and pepper to taste

Instructions:

1. Rinse shirataki noodles, boil for 2 minutes, and dry in a pan.
2. Brown turkey sausage in a skillet, then set aside.
3. Melt butter in the skillet, cook spinach until wilted, and add cream, Parmesan, and red pepper flakes.
4. Toss in noodles and sausage, heat through, and season with salt and pepper.

Nutritional Facts (Per Serving): Calories: 496 | Carbs: 10g | Protein: 19g | Fat: 13g | Fiber: 7g | Sodium: 550mg | Sugars: 6g

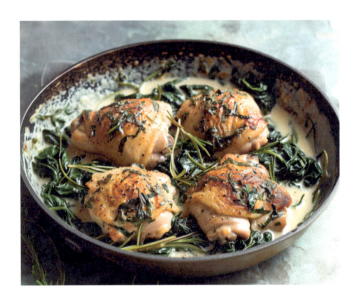

Rosemary Chicken Thighs with Creamy Spinach

Prep: 10 minutes | Cook: 20 minutes | Serves: 1

Ingredients:

- 2 bone-in, skin-on chicken thighs (300g)
- 1 tbsp olive oil (14g)
- 1/2 tsp dried rosemary (1g)
- 1 cup fresh spinach (30g)
- 1/4 cup heavy cream (60ml)
- 1 clove garlic, minced (5g)
- Salt and pepper to taste

Instructions:

1. Heat oil in a skillet over medium heat. Season chicken thighs with rosemary, salt, and pepper.
2. Cook skin-side down for 8–10 minutes, flip, and cook another 8–10 minutes until done.
3. Let rest 5 minutes. In the same skillet, sauté garlic, cook spinach until wilted, and stir in cream until thickened.
4. Serve chicken with creamy spinach, garnished with lemon if desired.

Nutritional Facts (Per Serving): Calories: 499 | Carbs: 8g | Protein: 18g | Fat: 13g | Fiber: 7g | Sodium: 530mg | Sugars: 6g

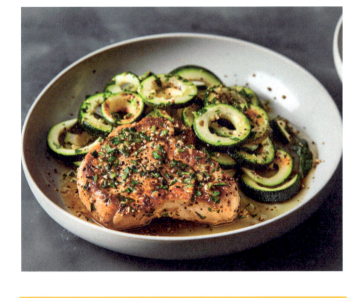

Herb-Crusted Pork Chops with Zucchini Ribbons

Prep: 10 minutes | Cook: 15 minutes | Serves: 1

Ingredients:

- 1 boneless pork chop (200g)
- 1/2 tsp mixed dried herbs (thyme, oregano) (1g)
- 1 medium zucchini, peeled into ribbons (200g)
- 1 tbsp grated Parmesan cheese (5g)
- 1 clove garlic, minced (5g)
- Salt and pepper to taste
- 1 tbsp olive oil (14g)

Instructions:

1. Heat olive oil in a skillet over medium heat.
2. Season pork chop with herbs, salt, and pepper, and cook 6–7 minutes per side until golden and 145°F (63°C).
3. Let rest 5 minutes. Sauté garlic in the same skillet, cook zucchini ribbons for 2–3 minutes, and toss with Parmesan before serving.

Nutritional Facts (Per Serving): Calories: 497 | Carbs: 10g | Protein: 19g | Fat: 12g | Fiber: 7g | Sodium: 540mg | Sugars: 7g

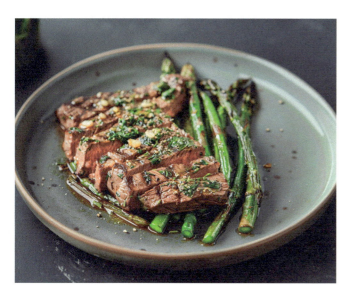

Garlic Butter Steak with Roasted Asparagus

Prep: 10 minutes | Cook: 15 minutes | Serves: 1

Ingredients:

- 6 oz ribeye steak (170g)
- 1 cup asparagus spears, trimmed (150g)
- 1 clove garlic, minced (5g)
- 1 tbsp butter (14g)
- 1 tsp olive oil (5ml)
- Salt and pepper to taste

Instructions:

1. Preheat oven to 400°F (200°C). Toss asparagus with olive oil, salt, and pepper, and roast for 10 minutes.
2. Heat a skillet over medium-high heat. Season steak with salt and pepper, and sear for 3-4 minutes per side for medium-rare.
3. Add butter and garlic to the skillet, spooning over the steak for 1-2 minutes.
4. Rest steak for 5 minutes, then serve with roasted asparagus.

Nutritional Facts (Per Serving): Calories: 500 | Carbs: 8g | Protein: 19g | Fat: 13g | Fiber: 7g | Sodium: 520mg | Sugars: 6g

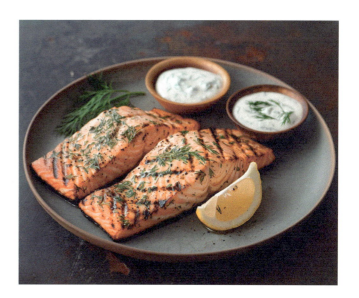

Grilled Salmon with Lemon Dill Sauce

Prep: 10 minutes | Cook: 10 minutes | Serves: 1

Ingredients:

- 6 oz salmon fillet (170g)
- 1 tbsp olive oil (14g)
- 1 tbsp chopped fresh dill (2g)
- 2 tbsp sour cream (30g)
- Salt and pepper to taste
- Juice of 1/2 lemon (15ml)

Instructions:

1. Preheat a grill or grill pan to medium-high and lightly grease with olive oil.
2. Pat the salmon dry, brush with olive oil, and season with salt and pepper. Place skin-side down on the grill and cook for 4-5 minutes without moving.
3. Flip and cook for another 4-5 minutes, or until it flakes easily. Rest for a few minutes.
4. Meanwhile, mix sour cream, lemon juice, dill, and salt in a bowl for the sauce. Mix until smooth and well blended.
5. Serve salmon with lemon dill sauce, garnished with capers or additional lemon wedges if desired.

Nutritional Facts (Per Serving): Calories: 496 | Carbs: 6g | Protein: 18g | Fat: 13g | Fiber: 7g | Sodium: 530mg | Sugars: 5g

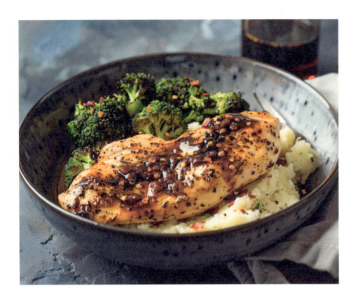

Balsamic-Glazed Chicken with Broccoli Mash

Prep: 10 minutes | Cook: 20 minutes | Serves: 1

Ingredients:

- 1 boneless, skinless chicken breast (200g)
- 1 tbsp olive oil (14g)
- 2 tbsp balsamic vinegar (30ml)
- 1 tsp low carb sweetener (4g)
- 2 cups broccoli florets (300g)
- 2 tbsp heavy cream (30ml)
- 1 tbsp butter (14g)
- Salt and pepper to taste

Instructions:

1. Heat olive oil in a skillet over medium heat. Season chicken, sear 5-6 minutes per side, and set aside.
2. Add balsamic vinegar and sweetener (or low-carb alternative) to the skillet. Cook for 2-3 minutes until reduced and slightly thickened, then coat chicken in the glaze.
3. Steam broccoli for 8 minutes, then mash with cream, butter, salt, and pepper until smooth.
4. Serve chicken over broccoli mash, garnished with additional glaze if desired.

Nutritional Facts (Per Serving): Calories: 498 | Carbs: 12g | Protein: 19g | Fat: 13g | Fiber: 7g | Sodium: 530mg | Sugars: 6g

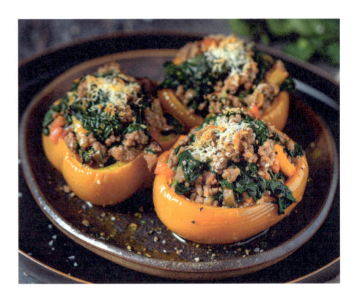

Stuffed Bell Peppers with Lamb and Spinach

Prep: 15 minutes | Cook: 25 minutes | Serves: 1

Ingredients:

- 1 large bell pepper, halved and seeded (150g)
- 4 oz ground lamb (120g)
- 1 cup fresh spinach, chopped (30g)
- 1/4 cup grated Parmesan cheese (25g)
- 1 tbsp olive oil (14g)
- 1 clove garlic, minced (5g)
- Salt and pepper to taste

Instructions:

1. Preheat oven to 375°F (190°C).
2. Drizzle halved bell peppers with olive oil, season, and bake for 10 minutes.
3. In a skillet, cook ground lamb until slightly browned. Add garlic and spinach, cooking until wilted.
4. Stir in half the Parmesan and stuff the mixture into the peppers.
5. Sprinkle with remaining Parmesan and bake for 10 minutes until golden. Garnish with feta cheese, if desired.

Nutritional Facts (Per Serving): Calories: 497 | Carbs: 10g | Protein: 18g | Fat: 12g | Fiber: 7g | Sodium: 540mg | Sugars: 7g

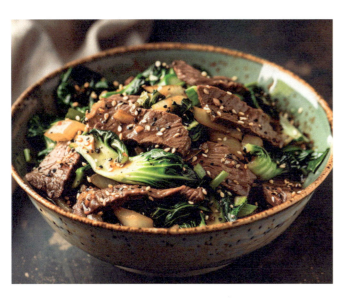

Sesame Ginger Beef with Bok Choy

Prep: 10 minutes | Cook: 15 minutes | Serves: 1

Ingredients:

- 6 oz flank steak, thinly sliced (170g)
- 1 tbsp grated fresh ginger (10g)
- 1 clove garlic, minced (5g)
- 2 tbsp soy sauce (30ml)
- 1 tsp low carb sweetener (4g)
- 2 cups baby bok choy, halved (300g)
- 1 tsp sesame seeds (5g)
- 1 tbsp sesame oil (14g)

Instructions:

1. Heat sesame oil in a skillet over medium-high heat. Add the sliced steak and sear for 3-4 minutes until browned. Remove and set aside.

2. In the same skillet, sauté ginger and garlic for 1 minute. Stir in soy sauce and low carb sweetener, cooking until slightly thickened.

3. Add bok choy to the skillet, tossing to coat in the sauce. Cook for 3-4 minutes until tender.

4. Return the beef to the skillet and toss with the bok choy. Sprinkle with sesame seeds and serve warm.

Nutritional Facts (Per Serving): Calories: 500 | Carbs: 10g | Protein: 18g | Fat: 13g | Fiber: 7g | Sodium: 540mg | Sugars: 6g

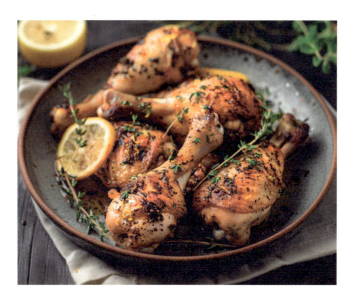

Crispy Chicken Drumsticks with Lemon and Thyme

Prep: 10 minutes | Cook: 35 minutes | Serves: 1

Ingredients:

- 2 chicken drumsticks (200g)
- 1 tbsp olive oil (14g)
- Juice and zest of 1/2 lemon (15ml)
- 1/2 tsp dried thyme (1g)
- 1 clove garlic, minced (5g)
- Salt and pepper to taste

Instructions:

1. Preheat oven to 400°F (200°C). Line a baking sheet with parchment paper.

2. Pat the chicken drumsticks dry with paper towels. In a bowl, combine olive oil, lemon juice, lemon zest, thyme, garlic, salt, and pepper. Toss chicken drumsticks in the mixture until well coated.

3. Place the drumsticks on the prepared baking sheet and bake for 30-35 minutes, turning halfway, until golden and crispy.

4. Serve hot, garnished with additional lemon zest, fresh thyme sprigs, and lemon wedges if desired.

Nutritional Facts (Per Serving): Calories: 495 | Carbs: 8g | Protein: 19g | Fat: 12g | Fiber: 7g | Sodium: 520mg | Sugars: 6g

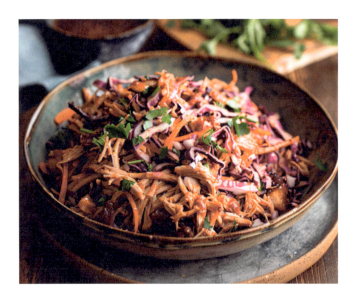

Keto BBQ Pulled Pork with Coleslaw

Prep: 15 minutes | Cook: 6 hours | Serves: 1

Ingredients:

- 6 oz pork shoulder, trimmed (170g)
- 1/4 cup low carb BBQ sauce (60ml)
- 1 tsp smoked paprika (2g)
- 1/2 tsp garlic powder (1g)
- 1/2 tsp onion powder (1g)
- Salt and pepper to taste
- 1 cup shredded cabbage (80g)
- 2 tbsp Greek yogurt (30g)
- 1 tsp apple cider vinegar (5ml)
- 1/2 tsp low carb sweetener (2g)

Instructions:

1. Season pork shoulder with smoked paprika, garlic powder, onion powder, salt, and pepper. Place in a slow cooker and cook on low for 6 hours or until tender. Shred the pork using two forks and mix with low carb BBQ sauce.
2. In a bowl, combine shredded cabbage, Greek yogurt, apple cider vinegar, low carb sweetener, salt, and pepper. Mix well to make the coleslaw.

Nutritional Facts (Per Serving): Calories: 497 | Carbs: 10g | Protein: 18g | Fat: 13g | Fiber: 7g | Sodium: 540mg | Sugars: 6g

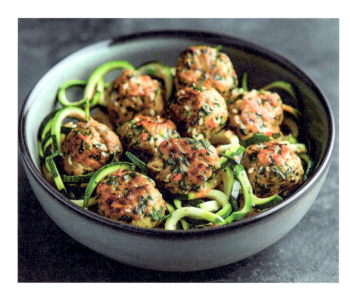

Turkey Meatballs with Pesto Zoodles

Prep: 15 minutes | Cook: 20 minutes | Serves: 1

Ingredients:

- 6 oz ground turkey (170g)
- 1 tbsp grated Parmesan cheese (5g)
- 1/2 tsp garlic powder (1g)
- 1/2 tsp dried oregano (1g)
- 1 tbsp olive oil (14g)
- 1 medium zucchini, spiralized (200g)
- 2 tbsp pesto sauce (30g)
- Salt and pepper to taste

Instructions:

1. In a bowl, mix ground turkey with Parmesan cheese, garlic powder, oregano, salt, and pepper. Form into small meatballs.
2. Heat olive oil in a skillet over medium heat. Cook one test meatball to check seasoning. Adjust the seasoning of the remaining mixture if needed.
3. Cook the meatballs for 10-12 minutes, turning occasionally, until golden and fully cooked. Remove and set aside.
4. In the same skillet, sauté zucchini noodles for 2-3 minutes until tender. Toss with pesto sauce.
5. Serve meatballs on pesto zoodles with basil.

Nutritional Facts (Per Serving): Calories: 494 | Carbs: 8g | Protein: 19g | Fat: 12g | Fiber: 7g | Sodium: 530mg | Sugars: 6g

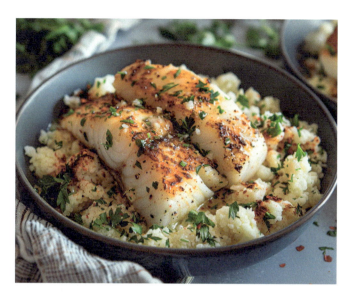

Pan-Seared Cod with Garlic Cauliflower Rice

Prep: 10 minutes | Cook: 15 minutes | Serves: 1

Ingredients:

- 6 oz cod fillet (170g)
- 1 tbsp olive oil (14g)
- 1 tsp garlic powder (2g)
- 2 cups cauliflower rice (300g)
- 1 tbsp butter (14g)
- 1 tbsp chopped fresh parsley (5g)
- Salt and pepper to taste

Instructions:

1. Heat olive oil in a skillet over medium heat. Season cod fillet with garlic powder, salt, and pepper. Cook for 3-4 minutes per side until golden and cooked through. Remove and set aside.
2. In the same skillet, melt butter and add cauliflower rice. Sauté for 5-7 minutes until tender. Stir in parsley, salt, and pepper.
3. Serve the cod fillet over the garlic cauliflower rice.

Nutritional Facts (Per Serving): Calories: 498 | Carbs: 8g | Protein: 18g | Fat: 13g | Fiber: 7g | Sodium: 520mg | Sugars: 6g

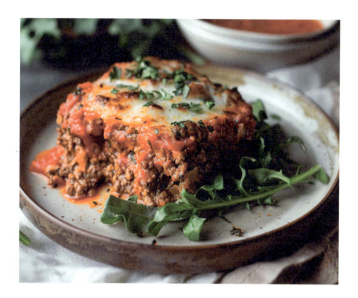

Italian-Style Meatloaf with Marinara and Mozzarella

Prep: 15 minutes | Cook: 40 minutes | Serves: 1

Ingredients:

- 6 oz ground beef (170g)
- 1 egg (50g)
- 1/4 cup grated Parmesan cheese (25g)
- 1 tsp dried Italian herbs (2g)
- 1/2 cup marinara sauce, no sugar added(120ml)
- 1/4 cup shredded mozzarella cheese(30g)
- Salt and pepper to taste

Instructions:

1. Preheat oven to 375°F (190°C). In a bowl, mix ground beef, egg, Parmesan cheese, Italian herbs, salt, and pepper until well combined.
2. Form the mixture into a small loaf and place on a baking sheet lined with parchment paper.
3. Bake for 30 minutes. Remove from the oven and top with marinara sauce and mozzarella cheese.
4. Return to the oven and bake for another 10 minutes, or until the cheese is melted and bubbly.

Nutritional Facts (Per Serving): Calories: 500 | Carbs: 12g | Protein: 19g | Fat: 13g | Fiber: 7g | Sodium: 540mg | Sugars: 6g

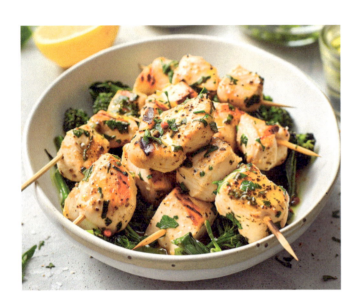

Lemon Garlic Chicken Skewers

Prep: 10 minutes | Cook: 15 minutes | Serves: 2

Ingredients:

- 1 lb chicken breast, cubed (450g)
- 2 tbsp olive oil (30ml)
- 2 cloves garlic, minced
- 1 tsp dried oregano (5g)
- 1/2 tsp salt (2.5g)
- 1/4 tsp black pepper (1g)
- Juice and zest of 1 lemon

Instructions:

1. In a bowl, mix olive oil, lemon juice, lemon zest, minced garlic, oregano, salt, and pepper.
2. Add chicken cubes to the marinade, toss to coat, and let sit for 15 minutes.
3. Thread chicken onto skewers.
4. Grill over medium heat for 12-15 minutes, turning occasionally, until chicken is cooked through.
5. Serve immediately with a side of vegetables or salad.

Nutritional Facts (Per Serving): Calories: 250 | Carbs: 8g | Protein: 23g | Fat: 6g | Fiber: 1g | Sodium: 320mg | Sugars: 4g

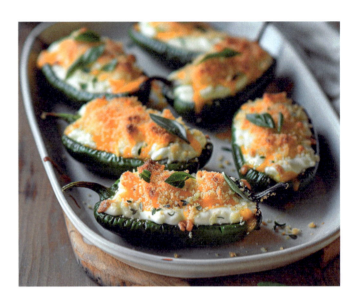

Baked Jalapeño Poppers with Cheddar Cheese

Prep: 15 minutes | Cook: 15 minutes | Serves: 2

Ingredients:

- 6 large jalapeños, halved and seeded (150g)
- 3 oz cream cheese, softened (85g)
- 1/4 tsp garlic powder (1g)
- 1/2 cup shredded cheddar cheese (60g)
- 1/4 tsp onion powder (1g)
- 2 tbsp almond flour (15g)

Instructions:

1. Preheat oven to 375°F (190°C). Line a baking sheet with parchment paper.
2. In a bowl, mix cream cheese, cheddar cheese, garlic powder, and onion powder.
3. Fill each jalapeño half with the cheese mixture.
4. Sprinkle almond flour over the tops for a crunchy texture.
5. Bake for 12-15 minutes until the tops are golden and bubbly.

Nutritional Facts (Per Serving): Calories: 252 | Carbs: 5g | Protein: 8g | Fat: 20g | Fiber: 2g | Sodium: 330mg | Sugars: 5g

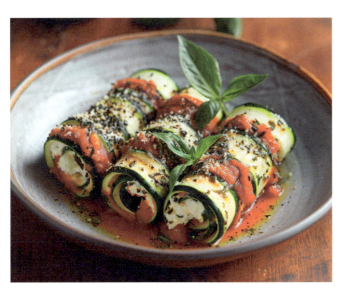

Zucchini Roll-Ups with Herbed Ricotta

Prep: 15 minutes | Cook: 10 minutes | Serves: 4

Ingredients:

- 2 medium zucchinis, thinly sliced lengthwise (400g)
- 1/4 cup grated Parmesan cheese (25g)
- 2 tbsp chopped fresh basil (8g)
- 1/2 tsp garlic powder (2g)
- Salt and pepper to taste
- 1/2 cup marinara sauce (120ml)
- 1 cup ricotta cheese (250g)

Instructions:

1. Preheat the oven to 375°F (190°C).
2. Lightly salt zucchini slices and let them sit for 5 minutes to remove excess moisture. Pat dry.
3. In a bowl, mix ricotta, Parmesan, basil, garlic powder, salt, and pepper.
4. Spread 1-2 tsp of the ricotta mixture onto each zucchini slice and roll tightly.
5. Place the rolls in a baking dish and top with marinara sauce.
6. Bake for 10 minutes until heated through.

Nutritional Facts (Per Serving): Calories: 247 | Carbs: 22g | Protein: 10g | Fat: 7g | Fiber: 2g | Sodium: 330mg | Sugars: 5g

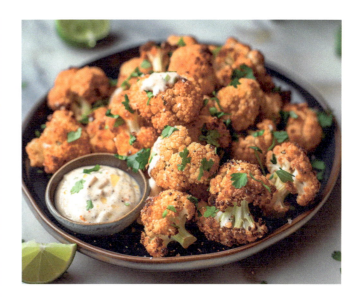

Crispy Cauliflower Bites with Garlic Aioli

Prep: 10 minutes | Cook: 20 minutes | Serves: 4

Ingredients:

- 1 medium cauliflower, cut into bite-sized florets (500g)
- 1/2 cup almond flour (60g)
- 1/4 cup grated Parmesan cheese (25g)
- 1 tsp smoked paprika (4g)
- 1/2 tsp garlic powder (2g)
- 2 large eggs, beaten
- Salt and pepper to taste
- 1 tbsp fresh parsley, chopped (5g)
- 1 tsp lemon juice (5ml)
- 1/2 tsp dried oregano (2g)
- Salt and pepper to taste

For Garlic Aioli:
- 1/4 cup Greek yogurt (60g)
- 1 clove garlic, minced
- 1 tsp lemon juice (5ml)

Instructions:

1. Preheat oven to 400°F (200°C) and line a baking sheet.
2. Mix almond flour, Parmesan, paprika, garlic powder, salt, and pepper in one bowl; place beaten eggs in another.
3. Dip cauliflower in egg, coat with almond mix, and bake for 20 minutes, turning once.
4. Mix mayo, garlic, and lemon for aioli.

Nutritional Facts (Per Serving): Calories: 245 | Carbs: 23g | Protein: 9g | Fat: 7g | Fiber: 3g | Sodium: 320mg | Sugars: 6g

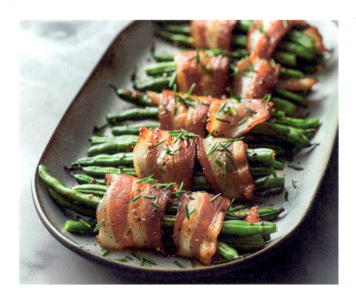

Bacon-Wrapped Green Beans

Prep: 10 minutes | Cook: 20 minutes | Serves: 4

Ingredients:

- 12 slices bacon (360g)
- 1 lb green beans, trimmed (450g)
- 1 tsp garlic powder (4g)
- Salt and pepper to taste
- 2 tbsp olive oil (30ml)

Instructions:

1. Preheat the oven to 400°F (200°C) and line a baking sheet with parchment paper.
2. Blanch green beans in boiling water for 3 minutes, then drain and pat dry.
3. Toss green beans with olive oil, garlic powder, salt, and pepper.
4. Bundle 5-6 green beans together and wrap with a slice of bacon. Secure with a toothpick if needed.
5. Arrange bundles on the baking sheet and bake for 18-20 minutes, turning once, until the bacon is crispy.

Nutritional Facts (Per Serving): Calories: 252 | Carbs: 20g | Protein: 10g | Fat: 7g | Fiber: 2g | Sodium: 330mg | Sugars: 5g

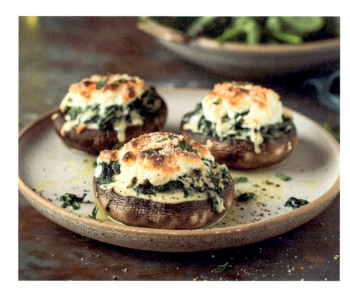

Stuffed Portobello Mushrooms with Spinach and Feta

Prep: 10 minutes | Cook: 20 minutes | Serves: 4

Ingredients:

- 4 large Portobello mushrooms (400g)
- 2 cups fresh spinach, chopped (60g)
- 1/2 cup crumbled feta cheese (75g)
- 1/4 cup grated Parmesan cheese (25g)
- 1 garlic clove, minced (5g)
- 1/4 tsp black pepper (1g)
- 1/4 tsp salt (1g)
- 2 tsp olive oil (10ml)

Instructions:

1. Preheat oven to 375°F (190°C).
2. Remove stems from mushrooms and brush caps with olive oil. Place on a baking sheet, gill side up.
3. Sauté spinach and garlic in a nonstick pan over medium heat for 2-3 minutes, until wilted.
4. Combine cooked spinach with feta, Parmesan, salt, and pepper.
5. Spoon the mixture evenly into the mushroom caps.
6. Bake for 15-20 minutes until the mushrooms are tender and the filling is golden.

Nutritional Facts (Per Serving): Calories: 246 | Carbs: 11g | Protein: 10g | Fat: 6g | Fiber: 2g | Sodium: 320mg | Sugars: 5g

CHAPTER 12: SNACKS: Flavorful Keto Sauces & Dips

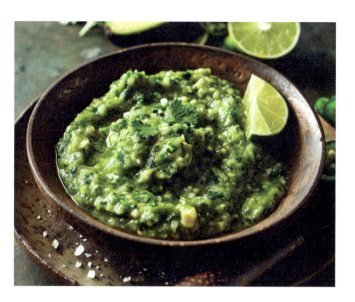

Avocado Lime Salsa Verde

Prep: 10 minutes | Cook: 1 minutes | Serves: 4

Ingredients:

- 2 ripe avocados, peeled and pitted (400g)
- 1/2 cup chopped fresh cilantro (20g)
- 1/2 cup chopped tomatillos (120g)
- 1 small jalapeño, seeded and finely chopped (10g)
- 2 tbsp lime juice (30ml)
- 1/4 tsp garlic powder (1g)
- Salt to taste

Instructions:
1. Place the avocados, cilantro, tomatillos, jalapeño, lime juice, garlic powder, and salt in a blender or food processor.
2. Blend until smooth and creamy, pausing to scrape down the sides as needed. Adjust salt to taste.
3. Transfer the salsa to a serving bowl. Chill in the refrigerator for 10 minutes to enhance the flavors.

Nutritional Facts (Per Serving): Calories: 249 | Carbs: 20g | Protein: 7g | Fat: 7g | Fiber: 2g | Sodium: 330mg | Sugars: 5g

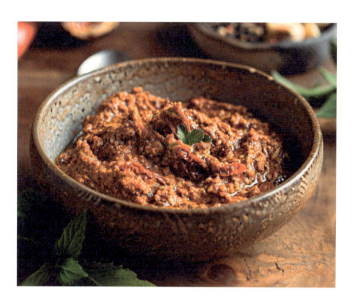

Sun-Dried Tomato and Walnut Spread

Prep: 10 minutes | Cook: 5 minutes | Serves: 4

Ingredients:

- 1/2 cup sun-dried tomatoes, packed in oil, drained (75g)
- 1/2 cup walnuts, toasted (60g)
- 1 garlic clove, minced (5g)
- 1 tbsp fresh lemon juice (15ml)
- 1/4 tsp salt (1g)
- 1/4 tsp black pepper (1g)
- 2 tbsp olive oil (30ml)

Instructions:

1. Place sun-dried tomatoes, walnuts, garlic, lemon juice, salt, and pepper in a food processor.
2. Pulse until the mixture is finely chopped.
3. While processing, slowly drizzle in olive oil until the spread reaches a smooth consistency.
4. Serve with low-carb crackers or vegetable slices.

Nutritional Facts (Per Serving): Calories: 247 | Carbs: 11g | Protein: 8g | Fat: 7g | Fiber: 2g | Sodium: 320mg | Sugars: 5g

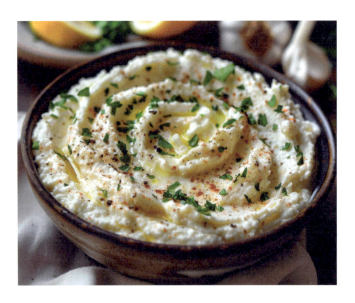

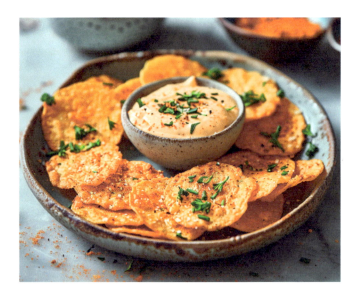

Lemon Garlic Yogurt Dip

Prep: 5 minutes | Cook: 1 minutes | Serves: 4

Ingredients:

- 1 cup plain Greek yogurt (240g)
- 1 tbsp lemon juice (15ml)
- 1 tsp lemon zest (2g)
- 1 clove garlic, minced
- 1 tbsp chopped fresh parsley (4g)
- 1/4 tsp salt (1g)
- 1/8 tsp black pepper (0.5g)

Instructions:

1. In a medium bowl, combine the Greek yogurt, lemon juice, and lemon zest. Mix well to ensure the yogurt absorbs the citrus flavor.
2. Add the minced garlic and stir thoroughly. For a smoother texture, use a whisk to incorporate the garlic evenly.
3. Fold in the chopped parsley and season with salt and pepper to taste. Adjust the seasoning if needed after tasting.
4. Cover the bowl and let the dip chill in the refrigerator for at least 10 minutes to allow the flavors to meld.

Nutritional Facts (Per Serving): Calories: 248 | Carbs: 10g | Protein: 9g | Fat: 6g | Fiber: 1g | Sodium: 330mg | Sugars: 5g

Smoked Paprika Mayo with Cheddar Crisps

Prep: 10 minutes | Cook: 10 minutes | Serves: 4

Ingredients:

- 1/2 cup Greek yogurt (120g)
- 1/2 tsp smoked paprika (2g)
- 1/4 tsp garlic powder (1g)
- 1 cup shredded sharp cheddar cheese (120g)

Instructions:

1. Preheat the oven to 400°F (200°C) and line a baking sheet with parchment paper.
2. Place 1 tbsp of shredded cheddar on the baking sheet, forming small mounds. Flatten slightly.
3. Bake for 6-8 minutes until golden and crisp. Cool completely.
4. In a small bowl, mix Greek yogurt, smoked paprika, and garlic powder until smooth.
5. Serve the mayo as a dip with the cheddar crisps.

Nutritional Facts (Per Serving): Calories: 251 | Carbs: 12g | Protein: 10g | Fat: 7g | Fiber: 1g | Sodium: 340mg | Sugars: 4g

CHAPTER 13: DESSERTS: Guilt-Free Low-Carb Treats

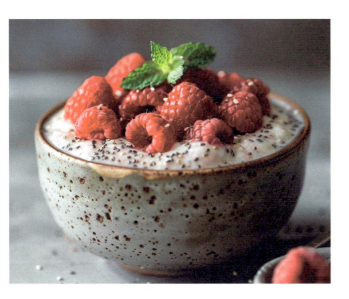

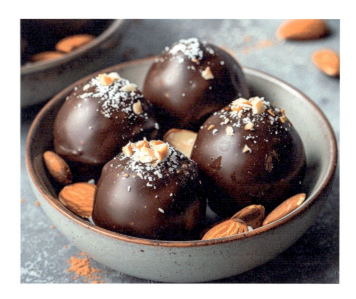

Coconut Raspberry Chia Pudding

Prep: 5 minutes | Cook: 1 minutes | Serves: 2

Ingredients:

- 1 cup unsweetened coconut milk (240 ml)
- 1 tbsp low-carb sweetener (15 g)
- 1/4 cup fresh raspberries (30 g)
- 1/4 tsp vanilla extract (1 ml)
- 3 tbsp chia seeds (40 g)

Instructions:

1. In a mixing bowl, whisk together coconut milk, chia seeds, low-carb sweetener, and vanilla extract until combined.
2. Let sit for 5 minutes, then whisk vigorously for 1 minute to prevent clumping.
3. Cover and refrigerate for at least 2 hours or overnight for the best texture.
4. Before serving, top each portion with fresh raspberries.

Nutritional Facts (Per Serving): Calories: 250 | Carbs: 18g | Protein: 8g | Fat: 6g | Fiber: 3g | Sodium: 320mg | Sugars: 6g

Dark Chocolate and Almond Keto Fat Bombs

Prep: 15 minutes | Cook: 5 minutes | Serves: 4

Ingredients:

- 1/2 cup dark chocolate (minimum 70% cocoa), chopped (80g)
- 1/4 cup almond butter (60g)
- 2 tbsp coconut oil (30ml)
- 1 tbsp low carb sweetener (15g)
- 1/4 cup chopped almonds (30g)

Instructions:

1. Gently melt chocolate, almond butter, and coconut oil over low heat until smooth.
2. Stir in the sweetener until fully dissolved.
3. Pour into small 1-inch molds, top with chopped almonds, and refrigerate for 1 hour or until firm.

Nutritional Facts (Per Serving): Calories: 249 | Carbs: 14g | Protein: 9g | Fat: 7g | Fiber: 2g | Sodium: 330mg | Sugars: 5g

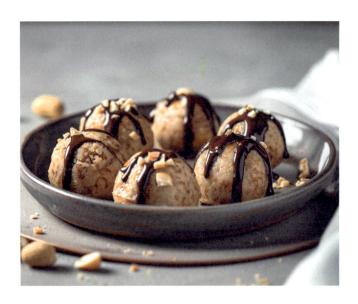

Sugar-Free Peanut Butter Cheesecake Truffles

Prep: 15 minutes | Cook: 1 minutes | Serves: 4

Ingredients:

- 1/2 cup cream cheese, softened (120g)
- 1/4 cup sugar-free peanut butter (60g)
- 2 tbsp low carb sweetener (30g)
- 1/4 tsp vanilla extract (1.25ml)
- 1/4 cup dark chocolate (minimum 70% cocoa), melted (40g)
- 1 tbsp chopped peanuts (15g)

Instructions:

1. Bring cream cheese and peanut butter to room temperature. Mix with sweetener and vanilla extract until smooth.
2. Scoop small portions and roll into bite-sized balls. Place the truffles on a parchment-lined tray and freeze for 15 minutes.
3. Dip in melted dark chocolate and sprinkle with chopped peanuts.
4. Refrigerate for at least 30 minutes before serving. Store in an airtight container in the fridge for up to 3 days.

Nutritional Facts (Per Serving): Calories: 245 | Carbs: 18g | Protein: 9g | Fat: 7g | Fiber: 2g | Sodium: 340mg | Sugars: 5g

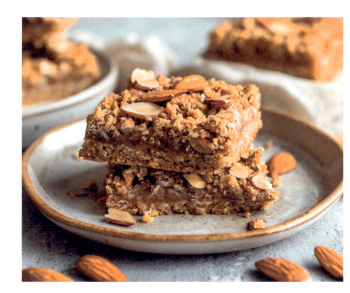

Cinnamon Almond Crumble Bars

Prep: 20 minutes | Cook: 25 minutes | Serves: 4

Ingredients:

- 1 cup almond flour (120g)
- 1/2 cup unsweetened shredded coconut (40g)
- 1/4 cup low carb sweetener (30g)
- 2 tbsp almond butter (30g)
- 1/4 cup melted butter (60ml)
- 1/2 tsp ground cinnamon (2g)
- 1/2 tsp vanilla extract(2.5ml)
- 1/4 cup sliced almonds(30g)

Instructions:

1. Preheat the oven to 350°F (175°C) and line an 8x8-inch (20x20cm) baking dish with parchment paper.
2. In a bowl, mix almond flour, shredded coconut, sweetener, melted butter, cinnamon, and vanilla extract to form a crumbly dough.
3. Press half the dough into the dish as the base. Spread room-temperature almond butter evenly over it.
4. Mix remaining dough with almonds, sprinkle over almond butter layer, and bake for 20–25 minutes until golden. Cool completely before cutting.

Nutritional Facts (Per Serving): Calories: 248 | Carbs: 18g | Protein: 8g | Fat: 7g | Fiber: 3g | Sodium: 330mg | Sugars: 6g

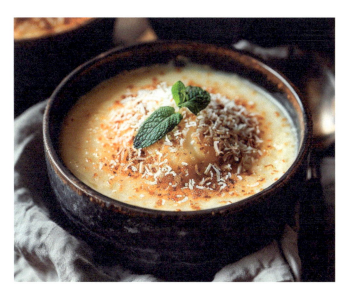

Keto Vanilla Coconut Custard

Prep: 10 minutes | Cook: 25 minutes | Serves: 4

Ingredients:

- 1 cup unsweetened coconut milk (240ml)
- 2 large eggs (100g)
- 2 tbsp low carb sweetener (30g)
- 1 tsp vanilla extract (5ml)
- 1/4 cup unsweetened shredded coconut (20g)
- 1/4 tsp salt (1g)

Instructions:

1. Preheat the oven to 350°F (175°C).
2. In a bowl, whisk together coconut milk, eggs, sweetener, vanilla extract, and salt until smooth.
3. Pour the mixture evenly into 4 small ramekins, filling each about three-quarters full. Sprinkle shredded coconut on top.
4. Place the ramekins in a baking dish and pour hot water into the dish until it reaches halfway up the sides of the ramekins (water should be 160-180°F/70-80°C).
5. Bake for 20–25 minutes until custard is set but slightly jiggly. Cool, then refrigerate for 1 hour before serving.

Nutritional Facts (Per Serving): Calories: 249 | Carbs: 12g | Protein: 8g | Fat: 7g | Fiber: 2g | Sodium: 330mg | Sugars: 6g

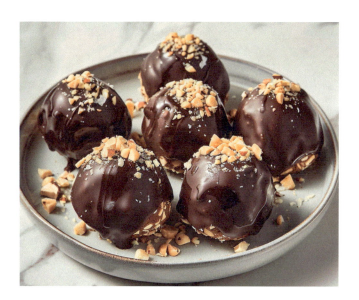

Espresso Chocolate Hazelnut Truffles

Prep: 15 minutes | Cook: 1 minutes | Serves: 4

Ingredients:

- 1/2 cup hazelnut butter (120g)
- 1/4 cup dark chocolate (minimum 70% cocoa), melted (40g)
- 1 tbsp coconut oil (15ml)
- 1 tbsp low carb sweetener (15g)
- 1 tsp instant espresso powder (2g)
- 2 tbsp finely chopped hazelnuts (30g)

Instructions:

1. In a bowl, mix hazelnut butter, melted dark chocolate, coconut oil, sweetener, and instant espresso powder until smooth.
2. Refrigerate the mixture for 15 minutes or until firm enough to shape.
3. Scoop small portions of the mixture and roll into truffle-sized balls. Roll each truffle in chopped hazelnuts to coat evenly.
4. Refrigerate 15 minutes before serving. Store in the fridge and serve with unsweetened coffee or tea.

Nutritional Facts (Per Serving): Calories: 250 | Carbs: 15g | Protein: 9g | Fat: 7g | Fiber: 3g | Sodium: 320mg | Sugars: 5g

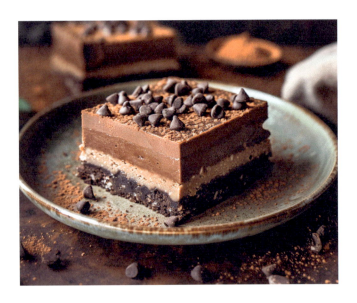

Keto Mocha Layer Bars

Prep: 20 minutes | Cook: 10 minutes | Serves: 4

Ingredients:

Mocha Layer:
- 1/2 cup dark chocolate (minimum 70% cocoa), melted (80g)
- 1/4 cup coconut cream (60ml)
- 1 tsp instant espresso powder (2g)

Base Layer:
- 1 cup almond flour (120g)
- 2 tbsp cocoa powder (15g)
- 2 tbsp low carb sweetener (30g)
- 1/4 cup melted butter (60ml)

Instructions:

1. Preheat the oven to 350°F (175°C). In a bowl, mix almond flour, cocoa powder, sweetener, and melted butter to form a dough.
2. Press the mixture into an 8x8-inch (20x20cm) pan lined with parchment paper and bake for 8-10 minutes. Let cool completely (approximately 15 minutes).
3. Mix dark chocolate, coconut cream, and espresso powder for the mocha layer. Spread over the cooled base.
4. Chill until set, then cut into bars.

Nutritional Facts (Per Serving): Calories: 248 | Carbs: 15g | Protein: 9g | Fat: 7g | Fiber: 2g | Sodium: 330mg | Sugars: 5g

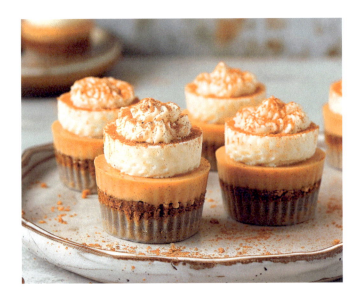

Spiced Pumpkin Cheesecake Cups

Prep: 15 minutes | Cook: 20 minutes | Serves: 4

Ingredients:

Filling:
- 1/2 cup pumpkin puree (120g)
- 1/2 cup cream cheese, softened (120g)
- 2 tbsp low carb sweetener (30g)
- 1/2 tsp pumpkin spice mix (2g)
- 1/4 tsp vanilla extract (1.25ml)

Crust:
- 1/2 cup almond flour (60g)
- 2 tbsp melted butter (30ml)
- 1 tbsp low carb sweetener (15g)

Instructions:

1. Preheat oven to 350°F (175°C). Mix almond flour, butter, and sweetener, then press into 4 cupcake molds for the crust.
2. Whisk pumpkin puree, cream cheese, sweetener, pumpkin spice, and vanilla until smooth.
3. Spoon filling over crusts and bake for 15–20 minutes.
4. Cool, then refrigerate for 1 hour before serving.

Nutritional Facts (Per Serving): Calories: 251 | Carbs: 18g | Protein: 8g | Fat: 7g | Fiber: 2g | Sodium: 320mg | Sugars: 6g

CHAPTER 14: DESSERTS: Celebration-Worthy Keto Sweets

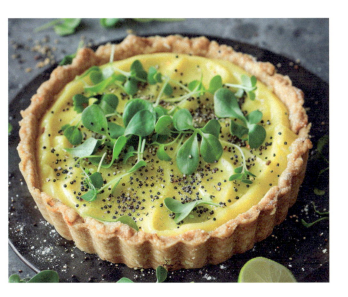

Sugar-Free Lime Tart

Prep: 20 minutes | Cook: 10 minutes | Serves: 4

Ingredients:

Filling:
- 1/2 cup heavy cream (120ml)
- 2 tbsp lime juice (30ml)
- 2 tbsp low carb sweetener (30g)
- 1/4 tsp vanilla extract (1.25ml)
- 1 tsp lime zest (2g)

Crust:
- 1 cup almond flour (120g)
- 2 tbsp melted butter (30ml)
- 1 tbsp low carb sweetener (15g)

Instructions:

1. Preheat oven to 350°F (175°C). Mix almond flour, butter, and sweetener, press into a tart pan, and bake for 8–10 minutes. Cool completely.
2. Whip cream with sweetener, lime, and vanilla. Spread over crust and chill 1 hour.

Nutritional Facts (Per Serving): Calories: 248 | Carbs: 12g | Protein: 7g | Fat: 7g | Fiber: 3g | Sodium: 320mg | Sugars: 5g

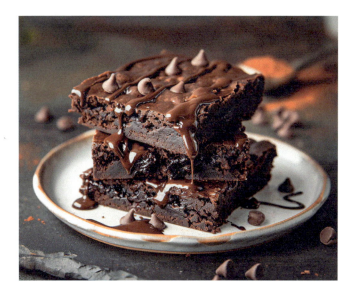

Almond Flour Chocolate Chip Brownies

Prep: 15 minutes | Cook: 20 minutes | Serves: 4

Ingredients:

- 1 cup almond flour (120g)
- 1/4 cup cocoa powder (30g)
- 1/4 cup low carb sweetener (30g)
- 1/4 cup melted butter (60ml)
- 2 large eggs (100g)
- 1/4 cup sugar-free chocolate chips (40g)
- 1/2 tsp vanilla extract (2.5ml)
- 1/4 tsp baking powder (1g)

Instructions:

1. Preheat oven to 350°F (175°C) and line an 8x8-inch dish.
2. Mix dry ingredients, then stir in butter, eggs, and vanilla. Fold in chocolate chips.
3. Bake for 18–20 minutes, cool, and slice.

Nutritional Facts (Per Serving): Calories: 246 | Carbohydrates: 3g | Protein: 5g | Fat: 22g | Fiber: 5g | Sodium: 130mg | Sugars: 0g

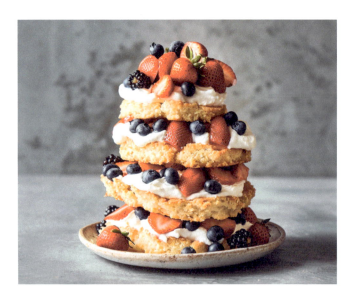

Strawberry Cream Keto Shortcake

Prep: 15 minutes | Cook: 20 minutes | Serves: 4

Ingredients:

- 1 cup almond flour (120g)
- 2 tbsp low-carb sweetener (25g)
- 1 tsp baking powder (5g)
- 2 large eggs (100g)
- 1 cup heavy cream (240ml)
- 1/4 cup melted butter (60g)
- 1/2 tsp vanilla extract (2.5ml)
- 1 cup sliced strawberries (150g)

Instructions:

1. Preheat oven to 350°F (175°C). Line a baking sheet with parchment paper.
2. In a bowl, mix almond flour, sweetener, and baking powder. Add eggs, melted butter, and vanilla extract, stirring until smooth.
3. Spoon batter onto the baking sheet to form 4 rounds, each about ½-inch thick. Bake for 15-20 minutes until golden. Cool completely.
4. Whip heavy cream with a little sweetener until fluffy. Slice the shortcakes in half, layer with whipped cream and freshly sliced strawberries, and top with the other half.

Nutritional Facts (Per Serving): Calories: 247 | Carbs: 8g | Protein: 8g | Fat: 6g | Fiber: 2g | Sodium: 310mg | Sugars: 5g

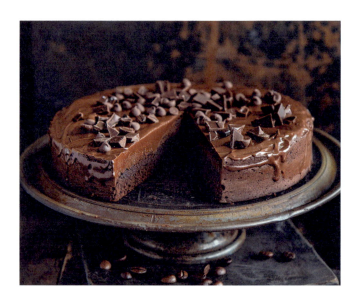

Rich Espresso Dark Chocolate Torte

Prep: 20 minutes | Cook: 25 minutes | Serves: 6

Ingredients:

- 1 cup almond flour (120g)
- 1/4 cup cocoa powder (30g)
- 1/3 cup low-carb sweetener (40g)
- 1 tsp baking powder (5g)
- 3 large eggs (150g)
- 1/4 cup melted butter (60g)
- 1 tsp vanilla extract (5ml)
- 2 tbsp brewed espresso (30ml)
- 1/4 cup dark chocolate chips (40g)

Instructions:

1. Preheat oven to 350°F (175°C). Grease a 6-inch (15cm) round cake pan and line with parchment paper.
2. In a bowl, sift almond flour and cocoa powder to remove lumps. Mix with sweetener and baking powder.
3. Whisk eggs, butter, vanilla, and espresso, then mix with dry ingredients until smooth. Fold in chocolate chips, pour into the pan, and bake for 20–25 minutes. Cool before slicing.

Nutritional Facts (Per Serving): Calories: 250 | Carbs: 15g | Protein: 9g | Fat: 7g | Fiber: 3g | Sodium: 320mg | Sugars: 6g

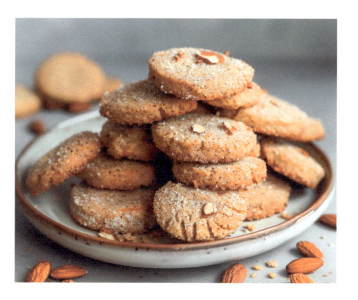

Keto Cinnamon Almond Cookies

Prep: 10 minutes | Cook: 15 minutes | Serves: 12

Ingredients:

- 2 cups almond flour (240g)
- 1/3 cup low-carb sweetener (40g)
- 1 tsp cinnamon (2g)
- 1/4 tsp salt (1g)
- 1/4 cup melted butter (60g)
- 1 large egg (50g)
- 1/2 tsp vanilla extract (2.5ml)

Instructions:

1. Preheat oven to 350°F (175°C) and line a baking sheet with parchment paper.
2. Mix almond flour, sweetener, cinnamon, and salt in a bowl.
3. Add melted butter, egg, and vanilla extract, stirring until dough forms.
4. Scoop dough into 12 balls and flatten slightly with your palm for even baking.
5. Bake for 12-15 minutes until golden. Let the cookies cool on the baking sheet for 10 minutes, as they will firm up upon cooling.

Nutritional Facts (Per Serving): Calories: 249 | Carbs: 9g | Protein: 8g | Fat: 6g | Fiber: 2g | Sodium: 310mg | Sugars: 5g

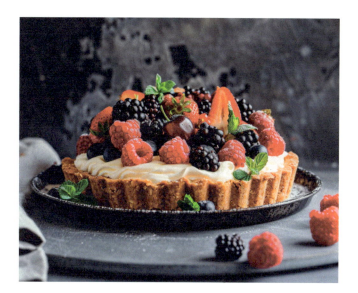

Fresh Berry Almond Flour Tart

Prep: 20 minutes | Cook: 15 minutes | Serves: 8

Ingredients:

- 2 cups almond flour (240g)
- 1/4 cup low-carb sweetener (30g)
- 1/4 cup melted butter (60g)
- 1 tsp vanilla extract (5ml)
- 2 cups fresh mixed berries (300g)
- 1 cup heavy cream (240ml)

Instructions:

1. Preheat oven to 350°F (175°C). Grease a tart pan.
2. Mix almond flour, sweetener, and melted butter until combined. Press the mixture evenly into the tart pan, ensuring a consistent thickness. Bake for 10-12 minutes until lightly golden, then cool completely.
3. Whip heavy cream with a little sweetener and vanilla extract until stiff peaks form.
4. Spread whipped cream over the cooled crust and top with fresh mixed berries. Chill before serving.

Nutritional Facts (Per Serving): Calories: 246 | Carbs: 15g | Protein: 9g | Fat: 7g | Fiber: 4g | Sodium: 320mg | Sugars: 6g

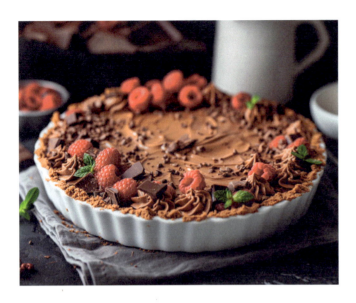

Decadent Dark Chocolate Mousse Pie

Prep: 15 minutes | Cook: 20 minutes | Serves: 8

Ingredients:

- 1 1/2 cups almond flour (180g)
- 1/4 cup cocoa powder (30g)
- 1/3 cup low-carb sweetener (40g)
- 1/4 cup melted butter (60g)
- 1 1/2 cups heavy cream (360ml)
- 1/2 cup dark chocolate chips (80g)
- 1 tsp vanilla extract (5ml)

Instructions:

1. Preheat oven to 350°F (175°C). Mix almond flour, cocoa powder, sweetener, and melted butter until combined. Press into a pie pan and bake for 8-10 minutes. Cool completely.
2. Melt chocolate chips in a double boiler or microwave in 30-second intervals, stirring until smooth.
3. Whip heavy cream with vanilla extract until stiff peaks form. Fold in melted chocolate until fully combined.
4. Spread the mousse over the cooled crust.

Nutritional Facts (Per Serving): Calories: 250 | Carbs: 18g | Protein: 8g | Fat: 6g | Fiber: 5g | Sodium: 320mg | Sugars: 6g

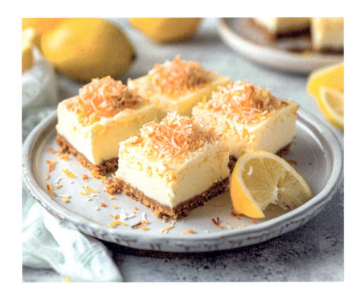

Lemon Coconut Cheesecake Squares

Prep: 20 minutes | Cook: 25 minutes | Serves: 9

Ingredients:

- 1 cup almond flour (120g)
- 1/3 cup shredded coconut (40g)
- 2 tbsp low-carb sweetener (25g)
- 8 oz cream cheese (225g)
- 2 large eggs (100g)
- 1/4 cup lemon juice (60ml)
- 1 tsp lemon zest (2g)
- 1/4 cup low-carb sweetener (30g)
- 1/4 cup melted butter (60g)

Instructions:

1. Preheat oven to 350°F (175°C). Mix almond flour, shredded coconut, melted butter, and sweetener. Press the mixture into a baking dish and bake for 8-10 minutes until golden.
2. In a mixing bowl, whisk cream cheese, eggs, lemon juice, zest, and sweetener until smooth and lump-free.
3. Pour the filling over the crust and bake for 15-18 minutes until set. Cool to room temperature, then chill for 1 hour. Cut into squares using a sharp knife for clean edges.

Nutritional Facts (Per Serving): Calories: 249 | Carbs: 13g | Protein: 9g | Fat: 7g | Fiber: 3g | Sodium: 330mg | Sugars: 5g

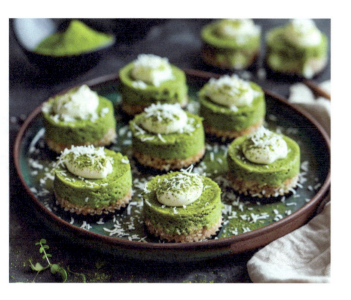

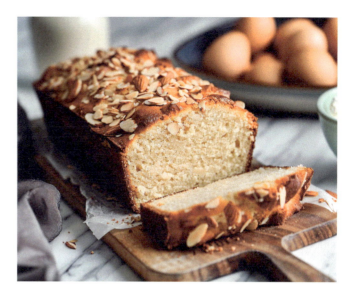

Matcha Coconut Keto Cheesecake Bites

Prep: 15 minutes | Cook: 20 minutes | Serves: 12

Ingredients:

- 1 1/2 cups almond flour (180g)
- 1/4 cup shredded coconut (30g)
- 1/4 cup melted butter (60g)
- 2 tbsp low-carb sweetener (25g)
- 8 oz cream cheese (225g)
- 1 large egg (50g)
- 1/4 cup heavy cream (60ml)
- 1 tsp matcha powder (2g)
- 1/4 cup low-carb sweetener (30g)

Instructions:

1. Preheat oven to 350°F (175°C). Mix almond flour, shredded coconut, melted butter, and sweetener. Press the mixture into a standard 12-cup muffin tin to form crusts. Bake for 8-10 minutes until golden.
2. Blend cream cheese, egg, heavy cream, matcha powder, and sweetener using a food processor or hand mixer until smooth.
3. Spoon the filling evenly onto the crusts. Bake for 10-12 minutes until set.

Nutritional Facts (Per Serving): Calories: 250 | Carbs: 13g | Protein: 9g | Fat: 7g | Fiber: 3g | Sodium: 320mg | Sugars: 5g

Keto Ricotta Almond Pound Cake

Prep: 10 minutes | Cook: 50 minutes | Serves: 10

Ingredients:

- 2 cups almond flour (240g)
- 1/2 tsp baking powder (2g)
- 1/4 cup low-carb sweetener (30g)
- 1/2 cup ricotta cheese (120g)
- 1/4 cup melted butter (60g)
- 1 tsp vanilla extract (5ml)
- 1/2 tsp almond extract (2.5ml)
- 3 large eggs (150g)

Instructions:

1. Preheat oven to 350°F (175°C). Grease a loaf pan and line it with parchment paper for easy removal.
2. Mix almond flour, baking powder, and sweetener in a bowl.
3. In another bowl, whisk eggs, ricotta cheese, melted butter, vanilla extract, and almond extract until smooth. Combine with dry ingredients.
4. Pour the batter into the prepared loaf pan and bake for 45-50 minutes. Check doneness by inserting a toothpick into the center it should come out clean. Cool completely before slicing.

Nutritional Facts (Per Serving): Calories: 247 | Carbs: 12g | Protein: 10g | Fat: 6g | Fiber: 2g | Sodium: 330mg | Sugars: 6g

CHAPTER 15: DINNER: Quick & Easy Keto Dinner Recipes

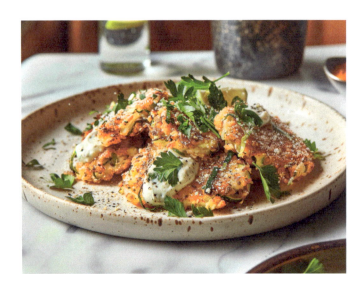

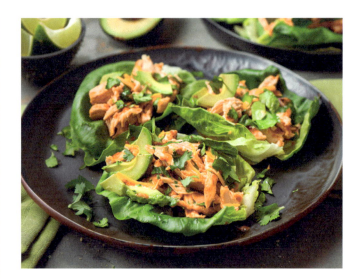

Parmesan-Crusted Zucchini Fritters with Lemon Yogurt Sauce

Prep: 10 minutes | Cook: 10 minutes | Serves: 2

Ingredients:

- 1 medium zucchini, grated (200g)
- 1/4 cup grated Parmesan (25g)
- 1/4 cup almond flour (25g)
- 1 egg (50g)
- 1/2 tsp garlic powder (2g)
- 1 tbsp olive oil (15ml)

Lemon Yogurt Sauce:
- 1/2 cup plain Greek yogurt (120g)
- 1 tbsp fresh lemon juice (15ml)

Instructions:

1. Squeeze zucchini to remove water.
2. Mix with Parmesan, almond flour, egg, and garlic powder. Fry fritters in oil for 2 minutes per side.
3. Mix yogurt, lemon juice, and salt for sauce. Serve with fritters.

Nutritional Facts (Per Serving): Calories: 497 | Carbs: 18g | Protein: 16g | Fat: 12g | Fiber: 6g | Sodium: 450mg | Sugars: 6g

Chicken Avocado Lettuce Wraps with Cilantro Lime Dressing

Prep: 15 minutes | Cook: 10 minutes | Serves: 2

Ingredients:

- 1 cup cooked shredded chicken (150g)
- 1/2 avocado, sliced (75g)
- 4 large butter lettuce leaves (40g)
- 1/4 cup diced red bell pepper (35g)
- 1/4 cup shredded cheddar cheese (25g)

Cilantro Lime Dressing:
- 2 tbsp olive oil (30ml)
- 1 tbsp lime juice (15ml)
- 1 tbsp chopped fresh cilantro (5g)
- 1/4 tsp garlic powder (1g)
- 1/4 tsp salt (1g)

Instructions:

1. Combine chicken, avocado, bell pepper, and cheese. Whisk olive oil, lime juice, cilantro, garlic powder, and salt to make dressing.
2. Fill lettuce leaves and drizzle with dressing.

Nutritional Facts (Per Serving): Calories: 500 | Carbs: 18g | Protein: 16g | Fat: 9g | Fiber: 6g | Sodium: 450mg | Sugars: 6g

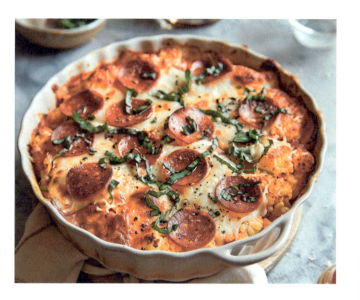

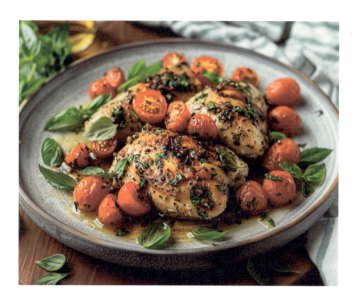

Cheesy Cauliflower Pizza Bake with Pepperoni

Prep: 15 minutes | Cook: 25 minutes | Serves: 2

Ingredients:

- 2 cups riced cauliflower (300g)
- 1 cup shredded mozzarella cheese (100g)
- 1/4 cup grated Parmesan cheese (25g)
- 1/4 tsp garlic powder (1g)
- 1/2 cup low-carb marinara sauce (120g)
- 1/2 cup sliced pepperoni (50g)
- 1 large egg (50g)

Instructions:

1. Preheat oven to 400°F (200°C). Line a baking dish with parchment paper.
2. Mix cauliflower, 1/2 cup mozzarella, Parmesan, egg, and garlic powder. Press into the dish to form a crust and bake for 18-20 minutes.
3. Spread marinara sauce on top, sprinkle with remaining mozzarella, and layer with pepperoni.
4. Bake for another 10 minutes until cheese is melted and bubbly.

Nutritional Facts (Per Serving): Calories: 498 | Carbs: 18g | Protein: 16g | Fat: 12g | Fiber: 7g | Sodium: 500mg | Sugars: 6g

Garlic Herb Chicken with Roasted Cherry Tomatoes

Prep: 10 minutes | Cook: 20 minutes | Serves: 2

Ingredients:

- 2 medium chicken breasts (200g each)
- 1 tbsp olive oil (15ml)
- 1 tsp garlic powder (5g)
- 1 tsp dried Italian herbs (5g)
- 1/4 tsp salt (1g)
- 1/4 tsp black pepper (1g)
- 1 cup cherry tomatoes (150g)

Instructions:

1. Preheat oven to 400°F (200°C). Rub chicken with olive oil, garlic powder, herbs, salt, and pepper.
2. Heat a skillet over medium-high heat and sear chicken for 2 minutes per side.
3. Transfer chicken to a baking dish, add cherry tomatoes, and bake for 15-18 minutes until chicken is cooked through.
4. Serve chicken with roasted tomatoes and pan juices.

Nutritional Facts (Per Serving): Calories: 495 | Carbs: 10g | Protein: 19g | Fat: 13g | Fiber: 6g | Sodium: 450mg | Sugars: 5g

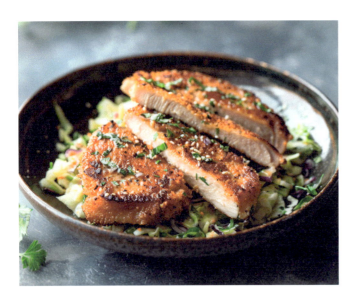

Crispy Pork Cutlets with Creamy Dijon Cabbage Slaw

Prep: 15 minutes | Cook: 15 minutes | Serves: 2

Ingredients:

- 2 boneless pork chops, pounded thin (200g each)
- 1/2 cup almond flour (50g)
- 1/4 cup grated Parmesan (25g)
- 1 large egg, beaten (50g)
- 1/4 tsp garlic powder (1g)
- 1/4 tsp salt (1g)
- 1/4 tsp black pepper (1g)
- 2 tbsp olive oil (30ml)

Cabbage Slaw:
- 2 cups shredded green cabbage (150g)
- 1/4 cup plain Greek yogurt (60g)
- 1 tbsp Dijon mustard (15g)
- 1 tsp apple cider vinegar (5ml)

Instructions:

1. Mix almond flour, Parmesan, garlic powder, salt, and pepper.
2. Dip pork chops in egg, then coat with the mixture. Fry in olive oil for 3–4 minutes per side until golden and cooked through. Rest 2 minutes.
3. Combine cabbage, yogurt, Dijon, vinegar, salt, and pepper for slaw. Serve pork with slaw.

Nutritional Facts (Per Serving): Calories: 501 | Carbs: 15g | Protein: 19g | Fat: 14g | Fiber: 7g | Sodium: 500mg | Sugars: 6g

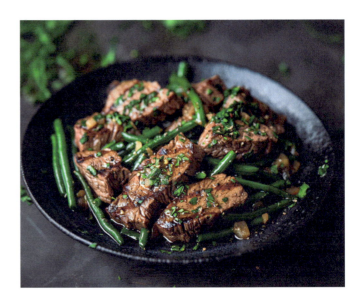

Seared Steak Bites with Garlic Butter Green Beans

Prep: 10 minutes | Cook: 15 minutes | Serves: 2

Ingredients:

- 8 oz sirloin steak, cut into bite-sized pieces (225g)
- 1 tbsp olive oil (15ml)
- 1 tbsp unsalted butter (15g)
- 2 cups trimmed green beans (150g)
- 1/4 tsp salt (1g)
- 1/4 tsp black pepper (1g)
- 1 tsp minced garlic (5g)

Instructions:

1. Heat olive oil in a skillet over medium-high heat.
2. Season steak bites with salt and pepper, then sear for 2-3 minutes per side. Remove from skillet and set aside.
3. In the same skillet, melt butter, add minced garlic, and sauté for 1 minute.
4. Add green beans to the skillet and sauté for 5-6 minutes until tender.
5. Return steak to the skillet and toss to combine. Serve immediately.

Nutritional Facts (Per Serving): Calories: 498 | Carbs: 12g | Protein: 19g | Fat: 12g | Fiber: 6g | Sodium: 450mg | Sugars: 5g

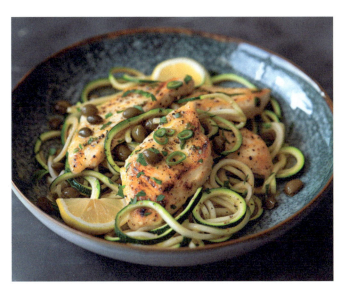

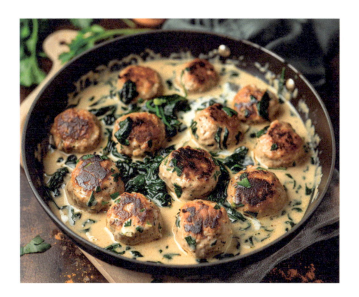

Lemon Chicken with Zucchini Noodles and Capers

Prep: 15 minutes | Cook: 20 minutes | Serves: 2

Ingredients:

- 2 medium chicken breasts (200g each)
- 2 tbsp olive oil (30ml)
- 1 tbsp fresh lemon juice (15ml)
- 1 tsp lemon zest (2g)

- 2 medium zucchinis, spiralized (300g)
- 1 tbsp capers (15g)
- 1/4 tsp salt (1g)
- 1/4 tsp black pepper (1g)

Instructions:

1. Heat 1 tbsp olive oil in a skillet over medium heat. Season chicken with salt and pepper and cook for 5-6 minutes per side until golden and cooked through. Remove and set aside.
2. Add remaining olive oil to the skillet, then sauté zucchini noodles for 2 minutes, ensuring they remain firm. Drain any excess liquid.
3. Stir in lemon juice, zest, and capers. Serve zucchini noodles topped with sliced chicken and pan juices.

Nutritional Facts (Per Serving): Calories: 499 | Carbs: 13g | Protein: 18g | Fat: 12g | Fiber: 7g | Sodium: 450mg | Sugars: 6g

Turkey Meatballs in Creamy Spinach Sauce

Prep: 15 minutes | Cook: 25 minutes | Serves: 2

Ingredients:

- 1/2 lb ground turkey (225g)
- 1/4 cup almond flour (25g)
- 1 large egg (50g)
- 1/4 tsp garlic powder (1g)
- 1/4 tsp salt (1g)
- 1/4 tsp black pepper (1g)

Spinach Sauce:
- 1 tbsp olive oil (15ml)
- 1/2 cup heavy cream (120ml)
- 1 cup fresh spinach, chopped (60g)
- 1/4 tsp nutmeg (1g)

Instructions:

1. Mix turkey, almond flour, egg, garlic powder, salt, and pepper. Form into small meatballs.
2. Heat olive oil in a skillet over medium heat. Cook meatballs for 8-10 minutes, turning occasionally, until browned and cooked through. Remove and set aside.
3. In the same skillet, add cream, spinach, and nutmeg. Cook for 2-3 minutes until spinach wilts. Return meatballs to the skillet and simmer for 2-3 minutes.

Nutritional Facts (Per Serving): Calories: 500 | Carbs: 9g | Protein: 17g | Fat: 14g | Fiber: 7g | Sodium: 500mg | Sugars: 5g

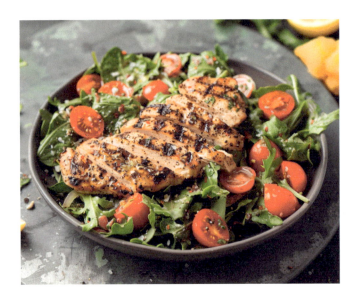

Grilled Chicken Salad with Lemon-Parmesan Dressing

Prep: 15 minutes | Cook: 15 minutes | Serves: 2

Ingredients:

- 2 medium chicken breasts (200g each)
- 1 tbsp olive oil (15ml)
- 6 cups mixed salad greens (300g)
- 1/2 cup cherry tomatoes, halved (75g)
- 1/4 cup grated Parmesan cheese (25g)

Dressing:
- 2 tbsp olive oil (30ml)
- 1 tbsp fresh lemon juice (15ml)
- 1 tsp Dijon mustard (5g)
- 1/4 tsp garlic powder (1g)
- 1/4 tsp salt (1g)

Instructions:

1. Grill seasoned chicken in olive oil for 6-7 minutes per side, slice, and set aside.
2. Combine greens, tomatoes, Parmesan, and dressing. Top with chicken.

Nutritional Facts (Per Serving): Calories: 499 | Carbs: 10g | Protein: 19g | Fat: 13g | Fiber: 7g | Sodium: 500mg | Sugars: 6g

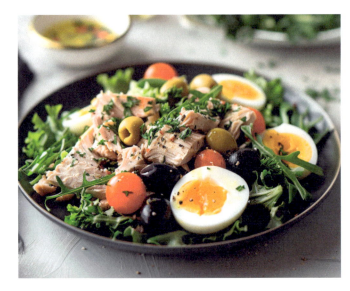

Keto Tuna Nicoise Salad with Olives and Eggs

Prep: 15 minutes | Cook: 10 minutes | Serves: 2

Ingredients:

- 1 can tuna in olive oil, drained (150g)
- 2 large eggs, hard-boiled and halved (100g)
- 2 cups green beans, blanched (150g)
- 1/4 cup black olives (40g)
- 4 cups mixed salad greens (200g)

Dressing:
- 2 tbsp olive oil (30ml)
- 1 tbsp red wine vinegar (15ml)
- 1 tsp Dijon mustard (5g)
- 1/4 tsp dried thyme (1g)
- 1/4 tsp salt (1g)

Instructions:

1. Arrange salad greens on plates and top with tuna, eggs, green beans, and olives.
2. Whisk together dressing ingredients and drizzle over the salad.

Nutritional Facts (Per Serving): Calories: 500 | Carbs: 12g | Protein: 18g | Fat: 12g | Fiber: 7g | Sodium: 500mg | Sugars: 5g

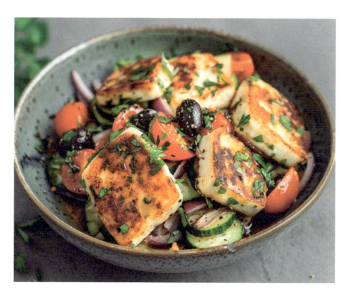

Greek Salad with Baked Halloumi and Fresh Herbs

Prep: 15 minutes | Cook: 10 minutes | Serves: 2

Ingredients:

- 8 oz halloumi cheese, sliced (225g)
- 2 tbsp olive oil (30ml)
- 2 cups chopped cucumber (300g)
- 1 cup cherry tomatoes, halved (150g)
- 1/4 cup sliced red onion (35g)
- 2 tbsp fresh parsley, chopped (10g)
- 1/4 cup black olives (40g)

Dressing:
- 2 tbsp olive oil (30ml)
- 1 tbsp red wine vinegar (15ml)
- 1/4 tsp dried oregano (1g)
- 1/4 tsp salt (1g)
- 1/4 tsp black pepper (1g)

Instructions:

1. Preheat oven to 400°F (200°C). Drizzle halloumi with olive oil and bake for 10 minutes, turning once.
2. Combine cucumber, tomatoes, onion, olives, and parsley.
3. Whisk olive oil, vinegar, oregano, salt, and pepper for dressing. Toss salad, then top with halloumi.

Nutritional Facts (Per Serving): Calories: 496 | Carbs: 12g | Protein: 16g | Fat: 13g | Fiber: 7g | Sodium: 500mg | Sugars: 6g

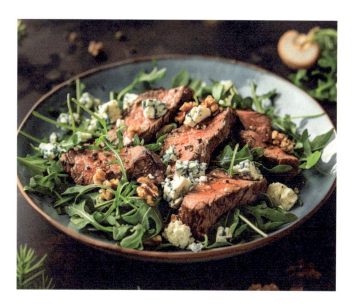

Warm Steak Salad with Arugula, Walnuts, and Blue Cheese

Prep: 15 minutes | Cook: 10 minutes | Serves: 2

Ingredients:

- 8 oz sirloin steak (225g)
- 2 tbsp olive oil (30ml)
- 4 cups arugula (200g)
- 1/4 cup crumbled blue cheese (30g)
- 1/4 cup chopped walnuts (30g)

Dressing:
- 2 tbsp olive oil (30ml)
- 1 tbsp balsamic vinegar (15ml)
- 1 tsp Dijon mustard (5g)
- 1/4 tsp garlic powder (1g)
- 1/4 tsp salt (1g)

Instructions:

1. Heat 1 tbsp olive oil in a skillet over medium-high heat. Season steak with salt and cook for 3-4 minutes per side until medium-rare. Let rest for 5 minutes, then slice thinly.
2. Arrange arugula on plates and top with steak slices, blue cheese, and walnuts.
3. Whisk together dressing ingredients and drizzle over the salad.

Nutritional Facts (Per Serving): Calories: 498 | Carbs: 10g | Protein: 18g | Fat: 13g | Fiber: 7g | Sodium: 500mg | Sugars: 5g

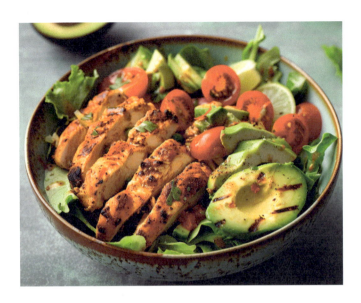

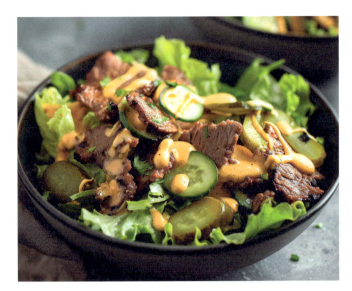

Spiced Chicken and Avocado Salad with Lime Dressing

Prep: 15 minutes | Cook: 15 minutes | Serves: 2

Ingredients:

- 2 medium chicken breasts (200g each)
- 1 tsp ground cumin (5g)
- 1 tsp smoked paprika (5g)
- 1 tbsp olive oil (15ml)
- 6 cups mixed salad greens (300g)
- 1/4 cup cherry tomatoes, halved (35g)
- 1/2 avocado, sliced (75g)

Dressing:
- 2 tbsp olive oil (30ml)
- 1.5 tbsp tbsp fresh lime juice (22ml)
- 1/4 tsp garlic powder (1g)
- 1/4 tsp salt (1g)

Instructions:

1. Rub chicken with cumin, paprika, and a pinch of salt. Heat olive oil in a skillet over medium heat and cook chicken for 5-6 minutes per side until fully cooked. Slice and set aside.
2. Arrange salad greens, avocado, and tomatoes in bowls.
3. Whisk olive oil, 1.5 tbsp lime juice, garlic powder, and salt to make the dressing. Drizzle over the salad and top with sliced chicken.

Nutritional Facts (Per Serving): Calories: 500 | Carbs: 12g | Protein: 18g | Fat: 14g | Fiber: 7g | Sodium: 500mg | Sugars: 6g

Classic Burger Salad with Pickles and Dijon Mayo

Prep: 15 minutes | Cook: 10 minutes | Serves: 2

Ingredients:

- 8 oz ground beef (225g)
- 1/4 tsp salt (1g)
- 1/4 tsp black pepper (1g)
- 4 cups chopped romaine lettuce (200g)
- 1/4 cup diced pickles (35g)
- 1/4 cup shredded cheddar cheese (25g)

Dressing:
- 2 tbsp Greek yogurt (30g)
- 1 tsp Dijon mustard (5g)
- 1 tbsp pickle juice(15ml)

Instructions:

1. Form ground beef into two evenly pressed patties and season with salt and pepper. Cook in a skillet over medium heat for 3-4 minutes per side until browned and cooked through. Crumble into pieces and set aside.
2. Arrange romaine lettuce, pickles, and cheddar cheese in bowls.
3. Mix mayo, Dijon, and pickle juice for dressing. Adjust with water or pickle juice if needed. Drizzle over salad and top with beef.

Nutritional Facts (Per Serving): Calories: 502 | Carbs: 10g | Protein: 17g | Fat: 13g | Fiber: 6g | Sodium: 500mg | Sugars: 5g

CHAPTER 17: DINNER: Keto Vegan Delights: Fresh & Flavorful

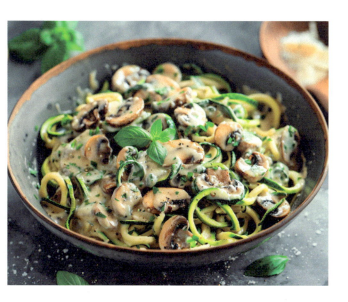

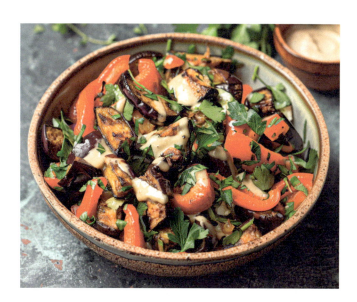

Zucchini Noodles with Vegan Alfredo Sauce and Mushrooms

Prep: 10 minutes | Cook: 10 minutes | Serves: 2

Ingredients:

- 2 medium zucchinis, spiralized (300g)
- 1 cup sliced mushrooms (150g)
- 1 tbsp olive oil (15ml)

Sauce:
- 1/2 cup almond milk (120ml)
- 2 tbsp cashew butter (30g)
- 1 tbsp nutritional yeast (15g)

Instructions:

1. Sauté mushrooms in olive oil for 5 minutes. Heat almond milk, cashew butter, nutritional yeast, salt, and pepper until thickened.
2. Toss zucchini noodles with mushrooms and sauce, and sauté for 2 minutes.

Nutritional Facts (Per Serving): Calories: 494 | Carbs: 20g | Protein: 14g | Fat: 12g | Fiber: 7g | Sodium: 450mg | Sugars: 6g

Roasted Eggplant and Bell Pepper Salad with Tahini Dressing

Prep: 5 minutes | Cook: 20 minutes | Serves: 2

Ingredients:

- 1 medium eggplant, diced (300g)
- 1 red bell pepper, diced (150g)
- 1 tbsp olive oil (15ml)
- 3 cups salad greens (150g)

Dressing:
- 1 tbsp tahini (15g)
- 1 tbsp lemon juice (15ml)

Instructions:

1. Roast eggplant and bell pepper with olive oil, salt, and pepper at 400°F (200°C) for 20 minutes.
Arrange salad greens in bowls, top with roasted vegetables.
Mix dressing ingredients and drizzle over the salad.

Nutritional Facts (Per Serving): Calories: 497 | Carbs: 15g | Protein: 12g | Fat: 13g | Fiber: 7g | Sodium: 450mg | Sugars: 6g

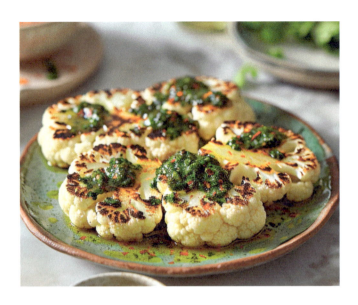

Cauliflower Steak with Chimichurri Sauce

Prep: 10 minutes | Cook: 25 minutes | Serves: 2

Ingredients:

- 1 large cauliflower, sliced into 1-inch steaks (600g)
- 2 tbsp olive oil (30ml)
- 1/4 tsp salt (1g)
- 1/4 tsp black pepper (1g)

Chimichurri Sauce:
- 1/4 cup fresh parsley, chopped (15g)
- 2 tbsp olive oil (30ml)
- 1 tbsp red wine vinegar (15ml)
- 1 tsp minced garlic (5g)
- 1/4 tsp chili flakes (1g)

Instructions:

1. Preheat oven to 400°F (200°C). Brush cauliflower steaks with olive oil, season with salt and pepper, and place on a baking sheet. Roast for 20-25 minutes, flipping halfway through.
2. In a bowl, mix parsley, olive oil, red wine vinegar, garlic, chili flakes, and a pinch of salt. Taste and adjust seasoning as needed.
3. Serve cauliflower steaks topped with chimichurri sauce.

Nutritional Facts (Per Serving): Calories: 499 | Carbs: 18g | Protein: 14g | Fat: 12g | Fiber: 7g | Sodium: 450mg | Sugars: 6g

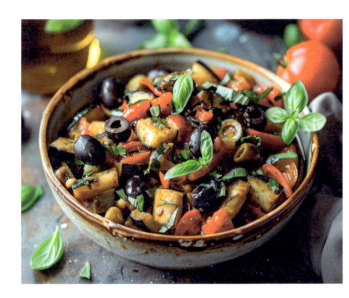

Vegan Ratatouille with Olives and Basil

Prep: 10 minutes | Cook: 30 minutes | Serves: 2

Ingredients:

- 1 medium eggplant, diced (300g)
- 1 red bell pepper, diced (150g)
- 1/2 cup diced tomatoes (120g)
- 1/4 cup black olives, sliced (40g)
- 2 tbsp olive oil (30ml)
- 2 tbsp fresh basil, chopped (10g)
- 1 zucchini, sliced (200g)

Instructions:

1. Heat olive oil in a large skillet over medium heat. Sauté eggplant for 5 minutes.
2. Add zucchini, bell pepper, and diced tomatoes. Stir well and cover. Simmer for 15-20 minutes, stirring occasionally, until vegetables are tender.
3. Stir in sliced olives and remove from heat. Sprinkle fresh basil over the ratatouille and drizzle with olive oil before serving.

Nutritional Facts (Per Serving): Calories: 500 | Carbs: 20g | Protein: 13g | Fat: 12g | Fiber: 8g | Sodium: 450mg | Sugars: 7g

CHAPTER 18: DINNER: Keto Seafood Delicacies

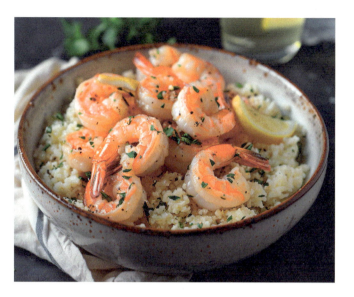

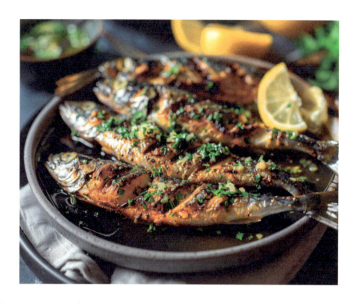

Shrimp Scampi with Lemon Garlic Cauliflower Rice

Prep: 10 minutes | Cook: 15 minutes | Serves: 2

Ingredients:

- 1 lb large shrimp, peeled and deveined (450g)
- 2 tbsp olive oil (30ml)
- 1 tsp minced garlic (5g)
- 1 tbsp fresh lemon juice (15ml)
- 1/4 tsp salt (1g)
- 2 cups riced cauliflower (300g)
- 1 tbsp chopped parsley (5g)

Instructions:

1. Heat 1 tbsp olive oil in a skillet over medium heat. Cook shrimp with 1/2 tsp garlic and a pinch of salt for 2-3 minutes per side until pink. Stir in 2 tsp lemon juice and set aside.

2. Sauté cauliflower rice in olive oil with salt and pepper for 5 minutes.

3. Serve shrimp over seasoned cauliflower rice, garnished with parsley.

Nutritional Facts (Per Serving): Calories: 501 | Carbs: 12g | Protein: 18g | Fat: 12g | Fiber: 7g | Sodium: 500mg | Sugars: 6g

Grilled Sardines with Lemon and Herb Oil

Prep: 10 minutes | Cook: 10 minutes | Serves: 2

Ingredients:

- 6 whole sardines, cleaned (300g)
- 2 tbsp olive oil (30ml)
- 1 tbsp fresh lemon juice (15ml)
- 1 tsp minced garlic (5g)
- 1 tbsp chopped fresh parsley (5g)
- 1/4 tsp salt (1g)

Instructions:

1. Preheat a grill to medium-high heat. Rub sardines with 1 tbsp olive oil and season with salt.

2. Grill sardines for 3-4 minutes per side until skin is crispy and fish is cooked through.

3. In a small bowl, mix the remaining olive oil, lemon juice, garlic, and parsley. Drizzle the herb oil over the grilled sardines before serving.

Nutritional Facts (Per Serving): Calories: 498 | Carbs: 10g | Protein: 14g | Fat: 12g | Fiber: 6g | Sodium: 450mg | Sugars: 5g

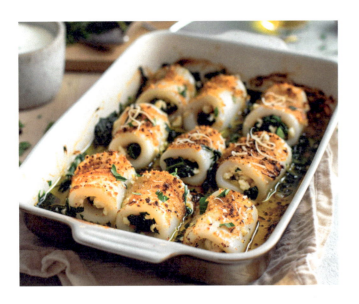

Baked Calamari Stuffed with Ricotta and Spinach

Prep: 15 minutes | Cook: 20 minutes | Serves: 2

Ingredients:

- 8 medium calamari tubes, cleaned (300g)
- 1/2 cup ricotta cheese (120g)
- 1/2 cup chopped spinach, cooked and drained (75g)
- 1 tsp minced garlic (5g)
- 1 tbsp olive oil (15ml)
- 1/4 tsp salt (1g)
- 1/4 tsp black pepper (1g)
- 1 tbsp grated Parmesan (15g)

Instructions:

1. Preheat your oven to 375°F (190°C) and lightly grease a baking dish with olive oil.
2. In a bowl, mix ricotta cheese, cooked spinach, Parmesan, garlic, salt, and pepper until smooth and well combined.
3. Stuff the ricotta mixture into the calamari tubes, filling them without overstuffing, and secure with toothpicks.
4. Arrange the stuffed calamari in the baking dish, drizzle with olive oil, and bake for 20 minutes, or until the calamari is tender and lightly golden.

Nutritional Facts (Per Serving): Calories: 500 | Carbs: 10g | Protein: 18g | Fat: 13g | Fiber: 6g | Sodium: 450mg | Sugars: 5g

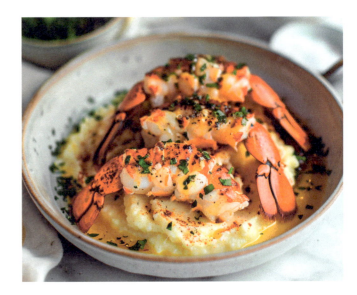

Butter-Poached Lobster with Cauliflower Puree

Prep: 15 minutes | Cook: 20 minutes | Serves: 2

Ingredients:

- 2 lobster tails (300g)
- 1/4 cup unsalted butter, melted (60g)
- 2 cups cauliflower florets (300g)
- 1/4 cup heavy cream (60ml)
- 1 tsp minced garlic (5g)
- 1/4 tsp salt (1g)
- 1/4 tsp black pepper (1g)

Instructions:

1. Steam cauliflower florets until tender, about 10 minutes.
2. Blend with heavy cream, garlic, salt, and pepper until smooth, adding more cream as needed to achieve the desired consistency.
3. Melt butter in a saucepan over low heat. Add lobster tails and poach for 5-6 minutes, basting frequently, ensuring the butter does not overheat or separate.
4. Serve poached lobster over the cauliflower purée and drizzle with the remaining butter.

Nutritional Facts (Per Serving): Calories: 502 | Carbs: 12g | Protein: 17g | Fat: 13g | Fiber: 7g | Sodium: 500mg | Sugars: 5g

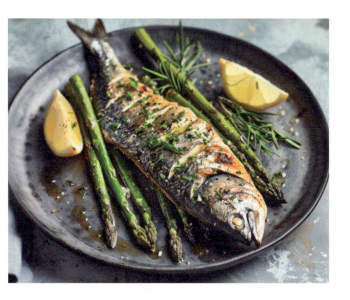

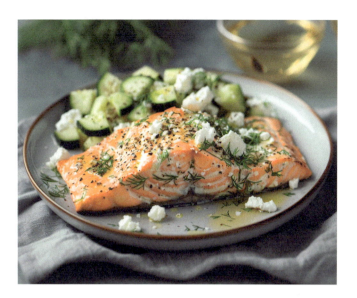

Mackerel in Lemon Herb Butter with Roasted Asparagus

Prep: 10 minutes | Cook: 20 minutes | Serves: 2

Ingredients:

- 2 whole mackerel, cleaned (400g)
- 2 tbsp unsalted butter, melted (30g)
- 1 tbsp fresh lemon juice (15ml)
- 1 tsp minced garlic (5g)
- 1 tbsp chopped parsley (5g)
- 1/4 tsp salt (1g)
- 1/4 tsp black pepper (1g)
- 1 lb asparagus, trimmed (450g)
- 1 tbsp olive oil (15ml)

Instructions:

1. Preheat oven to 400°F (200°C). Arrange asparagus on a baking sheet, drizzle with olive oil, and season with salt and pepper. Roast for 15 minutes until tender.
2. Mix melted butter, lemon juice, garlic, parsley, salt, and pepper in a small bowl. Brush the mixture over the mackerel.
3. Place mackerel on a baking sheet and bake for 15-18 minutes until cooked through. Serve with roasted asparagus, drizzled with remaining butter.

Nutritional Facts (Per Serving): Calories: 494 | Carbs: 9g | Protein: 19g | Fat: 13g | Fiber: 7g | Sodium: 450mg | Sugars: 5g

Dill-Crusted Salmon with Cucumber and Feta Salad

Prep: 15 minutes | Cook: 15 minutes | Serves: 2

Ingredients:

- 2 salmon fillets (200g each)
- 1 tbsp olive oil (15ml)
- 1 tbsp fresh dill, chopped (5g)
- 1 tsp Dijon mustard (5g)
- 1/4 tsp salt (1g)
- 1/4 tsp black pepper (1g)

Salad:
- 1 cucumber, sliced (200g)
- 1/4 cup crumbled feta cheese (30g)
- 1 tbsp olive oil (15ml)
- 1 tbsp fresh lemon juice (15ml)
- 1 tbsp chopped parsley (5g)

Instructions:

1. Preheat oven to 375°F (190°C). Brush salmon fillets with olive oil, then spread Dijon mustard over the top. Sprinkle with dill, salt, and pepper, pressing gently to adhere the dill. Bake for 12-15 minutes.
2. In a bowl, combine cucumber, feta, parsley, olive oil, lemon juice, salt, and pepper. Toss to coat.
3. Serve salmon with cucumber and feta salad on the side.

Nutritional Facts (Per Serving): Calories: 500 | Carbs: 12g | Protein: 17g | Fat: 13g | Fiber: 6g | Sodium: 450mg | Sugars: 5g

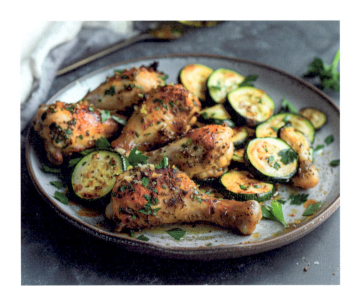

Lemon Herb Chicken Drumsticks with Zucchini Fries

Prep: 15 minutes | Cook: 30 minutes | Serves: 2

Ingredients:

- 6 chicken drumsticks (500g)
- 2 tbsp olive oil (30ml)
- 1 tbsp fresh lemon juice (15ml)
- 1 tsp minced garlic (5g)
- 1 tsp dried oregano (3g)
- 1/4 tsp salt (1g)
- 1/4 tsp black pepper (1g)
- 2 medium zucchinis, cut into fries (300g)
- 1/4 cup grated Parmesan (25g)

Instructions:

1. Preheat oven to 400°F (200°C). Pat chicken dry, toss with olive oil, lemon juice, garlic, oregano, salt, and pepper, and place on a baking sheet.
2. Slice zucchinis into fries, salt, let sit 10 minutes, and pat dry. Arrange on another sheet, sprinkle with Parmesan, and drizzle with olive oil.
3. Bake both trays for 25 minutes, flipping halfway, until chicken is cooked and fries are golden.

Nutritional Facts (Per Serving): Calories: 498 | Carbs: 14g | Protein: 18g | Fat: 13g | Fiber: 7g | Sodium: 450mg | Sugars: 5g

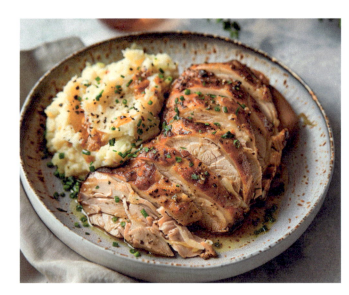

Slow-Cooked Pork Roast with Creamy Cabbage Mash

Prep: 15 minutes | Cook: 4 hours | Serves: 2

Ingredients:

- 1 lb pork shoulder roast (450g)
- 1 tsp smoked paprika (3g)
- 1/2 tsp garlic powder (2g)
- 1/4 tsp salt (1g)
- 1/4 tsp black pepper (1g)
- 1 tbsp olive oil (15ml)
- 2 cups chopped cabbage (300g)
- 1/4 cup heavy cream (60ml)
- 1 tbsp butter (15g)

Instructions:

1. Rub pork with paprika, garlic powder, salt, and pepper. Heat olive oil in a skillet over medium heat and sear pork for 2-3 minutes per side.
2. Transfer pork to a slow cooker and cook on low for 4 hours or until tender. Let rest for 10 minutes before shredding.
3. Steam cabbage until soft, then mash with heavy cream, butter, salt, and pepper until smooth.

Nutritional Facts (Per Serving): Calories: 501 | Carbs: 10g | Protein: 17g | Fat: 13g | Fiber: 6g | Sodium: 450mg | Sugars: 5g

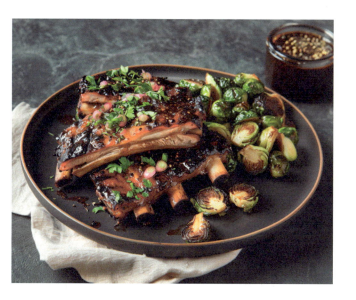

Smoky BBQ Ribs with Roasted Brussels Sprouts

Prep: 15 minutes | Cook: 2 hours | Serves: 2

Ingredients:

- 1 lb pork ribs (450g)
- 1 tsp smoked paprika (3g)
- 1 tsp garlic powder (3g)
- 1/2 tsp salt (2g)
- 1/2 tsp black pepper (2g)
- 1/4 cup low-carb BBQ sauce (60ml)
- 2 cups Brussels sprouts, halved (300g)
- 1 tbsp olive oil (15ml)

Instructions:

1. Preheat oven to 300°F (150°C). Trim excess fat from ribs and rub with smoked paprika, garlic powder, salt, and pepper. Wrap in foil and bake for 1.5 hours.
2. Increase oven temperature to 400°F (200°C). Unwrap ribs, brush with BBQ sauce, and bake for another 20-25 minutes until caramelized.
3. Toss Brussels sprouts with olive oil, salt, and pepper. Roast on a separate baking sheet for 20 minutes, stirring halfway through.
4. Serve ribs with roasted Brussels sprouts.

Nutritional Facts (Per Serving): Calories: 500 | Carbs: 14g | Protein: 18g | Fat: 12g | Fiber: 7g | Sodium: 450mg | Sugars: 6g

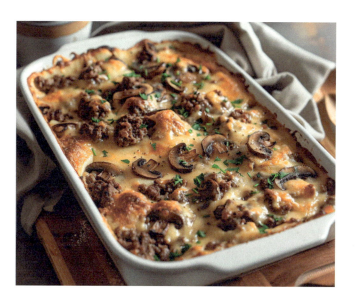

Beef and Mushroom Casserole with Almond Flour Crust

Prep: 15 minutes | Cook: 40 minutes | Serves: 2

Ingredients:

- 1/2 lb ground beef (225g)
- 1 cup sliced mushrooms (150g)
- 1 tsp garlic powder (3g)
- 1/4 tsp black pepper (1g)
- 1/2 cup shredded cheddar cheese (50g)
- 1/4 tsp salt (1g)

Crust:
- 1/2 cup almond flour (50g)
- 1 tbsp melted butter (15g)
- 1 large egg (50g)

Instructions:

1. Preheat oven to 375°F (190°C). Cook ground beef in a skillet over medium heat until browned. Add mushrooms, garlic powder, salt, and pepper, and sauté for 5 minutes.
2. Transfer beef mixture to a baking dish and sprinkle with cheddar cheese.
3. Mix almond flour, melted butter, and egg to form a batter. Spread batter evenly over the beef mixture.
4. Bake for 25-30 minutes until the crust is golden.

Nutritional Facts (Per Serving): Calories: 497 | Carbs: 12g | Protein: 17g | Fat: 13g | Fiber: 6g | Sodium: 450mg | Sugars: 5g

CHAPTER 20: BONUSES

30-Day Meal Plans with Shopping Guides: Simplified Keto Planning Made Easy

This cookbook features a handy 30-day shopping list specifically designed for the included recipes, all tailored to serve one person. It focuses on wholesome, high-quality ingredients that adhere to ketogenic guidelines, prioritizing healthy fats, low carbs, and minimal processed foods. Be mindful of hidden carbs in condiments, and feel free to adjust the quantities to fit your personal taste. Enjoy easy, flavorful keto meals and make your path to better health both enjoyable and stress-free!

Grocery Shopping List for 7-Day Meal Plan

Meat & Poultry

- **Chicken breast (boneless, skinless)** – 2 lb / 900 g (*Garlic Herb Chicken, Lemon Garlic Chicken Skewers*)
- **Ground lamb** – 1 lb / 450 g (*Stuffed Bell Peppers*)
- **Pork chops** – 1 lb / 450 g (*Crispy Pork Cutlets*)
- **Steak (sirloin or ribeye)** – 1 lb / 450 g (*Seared Steak Bites*)

Fish & Seafood

- **Salmon fillets** – 12 oz / 340 g (*Grilled Salmon*)
- **Shrimp (peeled and deveined)** – 1 lb / 450 g (*Shrimp Scampi, Keto Thai Coconut Shrimp Soup*)
- **Smoked salmon** – 8 oz / 225 g (*Eggs Benedict*)
- **Lobster tails** – 2 small (8 oz / 225 g) (*Butter-Poached Lobster*)

Vegetables

- **Zucchini** – 5 medium (*Zucchini Noodles, Zucchini Roll-Ups, Zucchini Pad Thai*)
- **Spinach (fresh)** – 3 bunches (*Ricotta-Stuffed Peppers, Spinach Smoothie, Stuffed Bell Peppers*)
- **Bell peppers (red or yellow)** – 4 medium (*Stuffed Peppers, Jalapeño Poppers*)
- **Cauliflower** – 2 heads (*Cauliflower Rice, Cauliflower Puree*)
- **Cherry tomatoes** – 2 pints / 600 g (*Garlic Herb Chicken*)
- **Brussels sprouts** – 1 lb / 450 g (*Garlic Butter Pork Bowl*)
- **Green beans** – 2 cups / 300 g (*Garlic Butter Green Beans*)
- **Jalapeños** – 4 medium (*Jalapeño Poppers*)
- **Garlic** – 1 bulb (*Various recipes*)
- **Onions (yellow)** – 2 large (*French Onion Soup*)

- **Herbs (fresh parsley, dill, basil)** – 1 bunch each (*Various recipes*)

Fruits

- **Lemons** – 6 large (*Hollandaise, Grilled Salmon, Shrimp Scampi*)
- **Avocados** – 3 large (*Egg Crepe Toast, Breakfast Bowls*)
- **Blueberries** – 1 pint / 300 g (*Antioxidant Shake*)
- **Raspberries** – 1 cup / 150 g (*Chia Pudding*)

Dairy & Eggs

- **Eggs** – 18 large (*Various recipes*)
- **Heavy cream** – 1 pint / 500 ml (*Hollandaise, Alfredo*)
- **Cheddar cheese (shredded)** – 8 oz / 225 g (*Egg Muffins, Jalapeño Poppers*)
- **Ricotta cheese** – 8 oz / 225 g (*Stuffed Peppers, Zucchini Roll-Ups*)
- **Gruyère cheese** – 6 oz / 170 g (*French Onion Soup*)

- **Parmesan cheese (grated)** – 4 oz / 110 g (*Alfredo, Garlic Butter Pork Bowl*)

Nuts, Seeds & Nut Butter

- **Chia seeds** – ½ cup / 75 g (*Chia Pudding*)
- **Almond flour** – 1 cup / 120 g (*Pork Cutlets, Custard*)

Pantry Staples

- **Olive oil (extra virgin)** – 1 bottle (*Various recipes*)
- **Butter (unsalted)** – 1 lb / 450 g (*Various recipes*)
- **Coconut milk (unsweetened, canned)** – 1 can (*Thai Shrimp Soup*)
- **Chicken stock** – 1 quart / 1 liter (*Soups, Alfredo*)
- **Coconut flour** – ½ cup / 60 g (*Custard*)
- **Salt, pepper, garlic powder, smoked paprika, dried thyme** – 1 jar each (*Various recipes*)

Meat & Poultry

- **Chicken thighs (boneless, skinless)** – 1.5 lb / 700 g (*BBQ Chicken Thighs, Balsamic-Glazed Chicken*)
- **Ground beef (80/20 lean)** – 1 lb / 450 g (*Keto Burrito Bowl*)
- **Turkey (ground)** – 1 lb / 450 g (*Savory Turkey Breakfast Meatloaf*)
- **Bacon** – 8 slices (*Pesto Mushroom and Bacon Bake*)
- **Beef steak (sirloin or ribeye)** – 12 oz / 340 g (*Warm Steak Salad*)

Fish & Seafood

- **Mackerel fillets** – 12 oz / 340 g (*Mackerel with Lemon Herb Butter*)
- **Sardines (fresh or canned)** – 10 oz / 280 g (*Grilled Sardines*)

Vegetables

- **Zucchini** – 6 medium (*Carbonara, Lemon Chicken, Zucchini Fritters, Zucchini Muffins*)
- **Spinach (fresh)** – 3 bunches (*Power Smoothie, Greek Egg Bake, Warm Salad*)
- **Cauliflower (heads)** – 2 large (*Cauliflower Rice, Broccoli Mash, Crispy Bites*)
- **Asparagus** – 1 bunch (*Mackerel with Roasted Asparagus*)
- **Tomatoes (medium)** – 6 (*Tomato Basil Soup, Tomato and Egg Boats, Ratatouille*)
- **Leeks** – 2 large (*Mushroom and Leek Stew*)
- **Mushrooms (white or cremini)** – 8 oz / 225 g (*Pesto Mushroom Bake, Mushroom Stew*)
- **Broccoli (florets)** – 1 head (*Broccoli Mash*)
- **Avocados** – 5 medium (*Smoothie, Burrito Bowl, Beef Burger*)
- **Lemons** – 5 medium (*Lemon Chicken, Sardines, Zucchini Fritters*)
- **Basil (fresh)** – 1 bunch (*Ratatouille, Tomato Soup*)
- **Garlic** – 1 bulb (*Various recipes*)

Fruits

- **Strawberries** – 1 cup / 150 g (*Keto Shortcake*)
- **Blueberries** – 1 cup / 150 g (*Berry Tart*)
- **Lime** – 2 medium (*Sugar-Free Lime Tart*)

Dairy & Eggs

- **Eggs** – 18 large (*Egg Bake, Breakfast Meatloaf, Egg Boats*)
- **Feta cheese** – 6 oz / 170 g (*Greek Egg Bake, Cauliflower Rice Bowl*)
- **Cheddar cheese (shredded)** – 8 oz / 225 g (*Zucchini Muffins, Beef Burger*)
- **Parmesan cheese (grated)** – 6 oz / 170 g (*Tomato Basil Soup, Zucchini Fritters*)
- **Blue cheese (crumbled)** – 3 oz / 85 g (*Warm Steak Salad*)
- **Cream cheese (full-fat)** – 8 oz / 225 g (*Mocha Layered Bars, Cream Tart*)
- **Heavy cream** – 1 cup / 250 ml (*Dark Chocolate Fat Bombs, Lemon Yogurt Sauce*)

Nuts, Seeds & Nut Butter

- **Almond flour** – 1.5 cups / 180 g (*Hash Browns, Tart Crust*)
- **Almonds (chopped)** – 1 cup / 150 g (*Fat Bombs, Crumble Bars*)
- **Walnuts (chopped)** – ½ cup / 75 g (*Warm Salad*)

Pantry Staples

- **Olive oil (extra virgin)**

– 1 bottle (Various recipes)
- **Coconut oil** – ½ cup / 120 ml (Fat Bombs, Crumble Bars)
- **Chicken stock** – 1 quart / 1 liter (Tomato Soup, Mushroom Stew)
- **Cinnamon** – 1 jar (Crumble Bars)
- **Cocoa powder (unsweetened)** – ¼ cup / 30 g (Mocha Bars)
- **Sugar substitute (erythritol or monk fruit)** – 1 cup / 200 g (Desserts)

Meat & Poultry

- **Chicken drumsticks** – 1.5 lb / 700 g (Lemon Herb Chicken)
- **Chicken breast (boneless, skinless)** – 1 lb / 450 g (Lentil Crepes, Zucchini Soup)
- **Ground beef** – 1 lb / 450 g (Beef Hash, Beef Waffle Sandwich)
- **Sausage (Italian, keto-friendly)** – 8 oz / 225 g (Spinach and Sausage Pasta)
- **Pork ribs** – 1 lb / 450 g (BBQ Ribs)
- **Pulled pork (pre-cooked or raw)** – 12 oz / 340 g (BBQ Pulled Pork)
- **Turkey breast (deli slices)** – 8 oz / 225 g (Turkey Wraps)
- **Bacon** – 8 slices (Bacon-Wrapped Green Beans)
- **Beef steak (sirloin or ribeye)** – 12 oz / 340 g (Garlic Butter Steak)

Fish & Seafood

- **Smoked salmon** – 8 oz / 225 g (Eggs Benedict)
- **Salmon fillets** – 12 oz / 340 g (Dill-Crusted Salmon)
- **Shrimp (peeled and deveined)** – 1 lb / 450 g (Shrimp Scampi)
- **Lobster tails** – 2 small (8 oz / 225 g) (Butter-Poached Lobster)

Vegetables

- **Spinach (fresh)** – 3 bunches (Waffles, Salad, Pasta)
- **Zucchini** – 6 medium (Zucchini Fries, Roll-Ups, Ribbons)
- **Cauliflower (heads)** – 2 large (Risotto, Cauliflower Puree)
- **Asparagus** – 1 bunch (Roasted Asparagus)
- **Bell peppers (mixed colors)** – 3 medium (Beef Hash)
- **Cucumber** – 2 medium (Cucumber Salad)
- **Brussels sprouts** – 1 lb / 450 g (Roasted Sprouts)
- **Mushrooms (white or cremini)** – 8 oz / 225 g (Risotto, Casserole)
- **Garlic** – 1 bulb (Various recipes)
- **Lemons** – 6 medium (Hollandaise, Lemon Dressing)
- **Sun-dried tomatoes** – ½ cup / 75 g (Spread)
- **Herbs (dill, parsley, thyme, basil)** – 1 bunch each (Various recipes)

Fruits

- **Pumpkin puree (canned)** – 1 small can

(Soup, Cheesecake Cups)
- **Limes** – 2 medium (Coconut Lime Shake)
- **Hazelnuts (roasted)** – ½ cup / 75 g (Truffles)

Dairy & Eggs

- **Eggs** – 18 large (Waffles, Eggs Benedict, Cookies)
- **Cheddar cheese (shredded)** – 8 oz / 225 g (Waffle Sandwich, Pasta)
- **Ricotta cheese** – 8 oz / 225 g (Zucchini Roll-Ups)
- **Feta cheese** – 6 oz / 170 g (Cucumber Salad)
- **Mozzarella cheese (fresh)** – 8 oz / 225 g (Turkey Wraps)
- **Cream cheese (full-fat)** – 8 oz / 225 g (Cheesecake Cups)
- **Parmesan cheese (grated)** – 6 oz / 170 g (Dressing, Risotto)
- **Heavy cream** – 1 cup / 250 ml (Hollandaise, Puree)

Nuts, Seeds & Nut Butter

- **Almond flour** – 2 cups / 240 g (Cookies, Brownies)
- **Almonds (chopped)** – ½ cup / 75 g (Brownies)
- **Walnuts (chopped)** – ½ cup / 75 g (Sun-Dried Tomato Spread)

Pantry Staples

- **Olive oil (extra virgin)** – 1 bottle (Various recipes)
- **Coconut oil** – ½ cup / 120 ml (Truffles, Brownies)
- **Chicken stock** – 1

quart / 1 liter *(Soup, Puree)*
- **Cinnamon** – 1 jar *(Cookies)*
- **Cocoa powder (unsweetened)** – ¼ cup / 30 g *(Truffles, Brownies)*
- **Sugar substitute (erythritol or monk fruit)** – 1 cup / 200 g *(Desserts)*

Grocery Shopping List for 22-28 Day Meal Plan

Meat & Poultry

- **Ground beef (80/20 lean)** – 1 lb / 450 g *(Burrito Bowl)*
- **Beef tenderloin** – 1 lb / 450 g *(Beef Tenderloin)*
- **Chicken breast (boneless, skinless)** – 1 lb / 450 g *(Grilled Chicken, Balsamic-Glazed Chicken)*
- **Pork ribs** – 1 lb / 450 g *(BBQ Pork Ribs)*
- **Chorizo sausage** – 8 oz / 225 g *(Breakfast Bowls)*
- **Bacon** – 8 slices *(Pesto Mushroom Bake, Crepe Toast)*
- **Turkey (ground or stew meat)** – 12 oz / 340 g *(Turkey Stew)*

Fish & Seafood

- **Mackerel fillets** – 12 oz / 340 g *(Mackerel with Lemon Herb Butter)*
- **Salmon fillets** – 12 oz / 340 g *(Dill-Crusted Salmon)*

Vegetables

- **Zucchini** – 6 medium *(Carbonara, Roll-Ups, Fritters)*
- **Spinach (fresh)** – 3 bunches *(Smoothies, Stew, Creamed Spinach)*
- **Bell peppers (red or yellow)** – 3 medium *(Eggplant Salad, Stuffed Peppers)*
- **Eggplant** – 1 large *(Eggplant Salad)*
- **Broccoli (florets)** – 1 head *(Broccoli Mash)*
- **Cauliflower (head)** – 1 large *(Casserole Crust, Parmesan Chips)*
- **Asparagus** – 1 bunch *(Garlic Butter Steak, Buttered Asparagus)*
- **Mushrooms (white or cremini)** – 8 oz / 225 g *(Pesto Mushroom Bake, Stew)*
- **Leeks** – 2 medium *(Mushroom Stew)*
- **Cucumber** – 2 medium *(Cucumber Salad)*
- **Garlic** – 1 bulb *(Various recipes)*
- **Lemons** – 6 medium *(Yogurt Sauce, Salad, Asparagus)*
- **Herbs (dill, parsley, basil)** – 1 bunch each *(Various recipes)*

Fruits

- **Avocados** – 5 medium *(Smoothies, Burrito Bowl, Crepe Toast)*
- **Raspberries** – 1 cup / 150 g *(Chia Pudding)*
- **Lime** – 3 medium *(Lime Tart, Sunrise Shake)*
- **Berries (mixed)** – 1 cup / 150 g *(Berry Tart)*

Dairy & Eggs

- **Eggs** – 18 large *(Egg Muffins, Crepe Toast, Fritters)*
- **Cheddar cheese (shredded)** – 8 oz / 225 g *(Egg Muffins, Burrito Bowl)*
- **Ricotta cheese** – 8 oz / 225 g *(Stuffed Peppers, Roll-Ups)*
- **Feta cheese** – 6 oz / 170 g *(Cucumber Salad)*
- **Cream cheese (full-fat)** – 8 oz / 225 g *(Pancakes, Cheesecake Cups)*
- **Parmesan cheese (grated)** – 6 oz / 170 g *(Tomato Soup, Fritters)*
- **Heavy cream** – 1 cup / 250 ml *(Mocha Bars, Lemon Yogurt Sauce)*

Nuts, Seeds & Nut Butter

- **Almond flour** – 2 cups / 240 g *(Tart Crust, Cookies)*
- **Almonds (chopped)** – ½ cup / 75 g *(Berry Tart)*
- **Hazelnuts (roasted)** – ½ cup / 75 g *(Truffles)*
- **Chia seeds** – ½ cup / 75 g *(Chia Pudding)*

Pantry Staples

- **Olive oil (extra virgin)** – 1 bottle *(Various recipes)*
- **Coconut oil** – ½ cup / 120 ml *(Truffles, Chia Pudding)*
- **Chicken stock** – 1 quart / 1 liter *(Stews, Mushroom Soup)*
- **Cinnamon** – 1 jar *(Cookies)*
- **Cocoa powder (unsweetened)** – ¼ cup / 30 g *(Mocha Bars)*
- **Sugar substitute (erythritol or monk fruit)** – 1 cup / 200 g *(Desserts)*

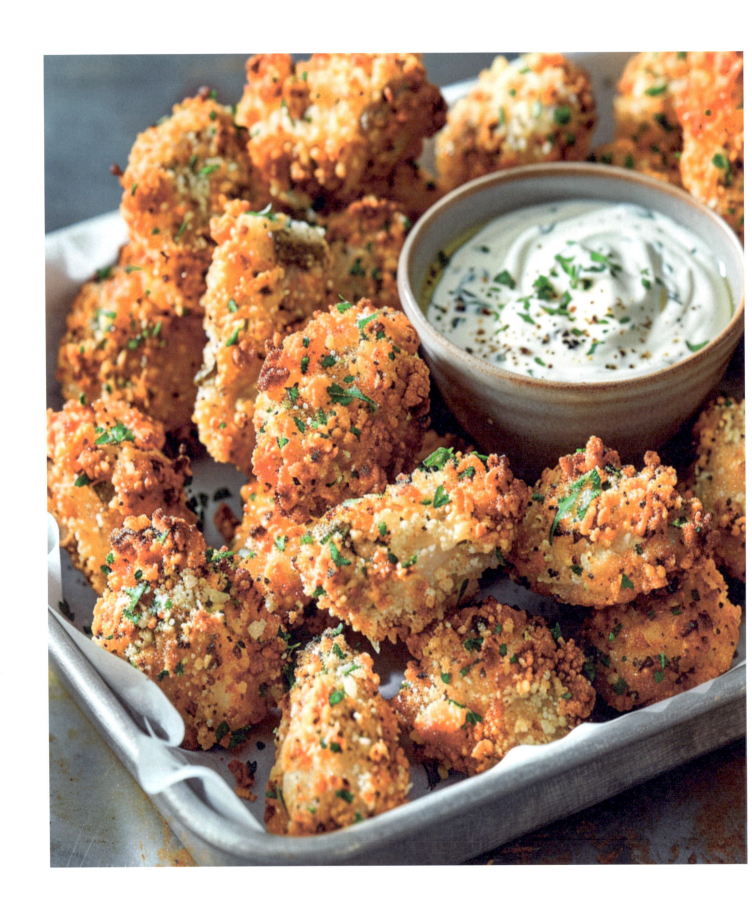

APPENDIX MEASUREMENT CONVERSION CHART

VOLUME EQUIVALENTS (DRY)

US STANDARD	METRIC (APPROXIMATE)
1/8 teaspoon	0.5 mL
1/4 teaspoon	1 mL
1/2 teaspoon	2 mL
3/4 teaspoon	4 mL
1 teaspoon	5 mL
1 tablespoon	15 mL
1/4 cup	59 mL
1/2 cup	118 mL
3/4 cup	177 mL
1 cup	235 mL
2 cups	475 mL
3 cups	700 mL
4 cups	1 L

US STANDARD	US STANDARD (OUNCES)	METRIC (APPROXIMATE)
2 tablespoons	1 fl.oz.	30 mL
1/4 cup	2 fl.oz.	60 mL
1/2 cup	4 fl.oz.	120 mL
1 cup	8 fl.oz.	240 mL
1 1/2 cup	12 fl.oz.	355 mL
2 cups or 1 pint	16 fl.oz.	475 mL
4 cups or 1 quart	32 fl.oz.	1 L
1 gallon	128 fl.oz.	4 L

TEMPERATURES EQUIVALENTS

FAHRENHEIT(F)	CELSIUS(C) (APPROXIMATE)
225 °F	107 °C
250 °F	120 °C
275 °F	135 °C
300 °F	150 °C
325 °F	160 °C
350 °F	180 °C
375 °F	190 °C
400 °F	205 °C
425 °F	220 °C
450 °F	235 °C
475 °F	245 °C
500 °F	260 °C

WEIGHT EQUIVALENTS

US STANDARD	METRIC (APPROXIMATE)
1 ounce	28 g
2 ounces	57 g
5 ounces	142 g
10 ounces	284 g
15 ounces	425 g
16 ounces	455 g
(1 pound)	680 g
1.5 pounds	907 g

VOLUME EQUIVALENTS (LIQUID)

Made in United States
Troutdale, OR
02/28/2025